PHARMACOLOGY - RESEARCH, SAFETY TESTING AND REGULATION

HEPARIN

STRUCTURE, DRUG DELIVERY APPLICATIONS AND CLINICAL OUTCOMES

PHARMACOLOGY - RESEARCH, SAFETY TESTING AND REGULATION

Additional books in this series can be found on Nova's website under the Series tab.

Additional e-books in this series can be found on Nova's website under the e-book tab.

PHARMACOLOGY - RESEARCH, SAFETY TESTING AND REGULATION

HEPARIN

STRUCTURE, DRUG DELIVERY APPLICATIONS AND CLINICAL OUTCOMES

NICOLE B. WILKINSON
EDITOR

NOVA BIOMEDICAL

New York

Library of Congress Cataloging-in-Publication Data

ISBN: 978-1-63117-624-1
LCCN: 2014935296

Published by Nova Science Publishers, Inc. † New York

Contents

Preface

Heparin is a highly sulphated glycosaminoglycan discovered about 90 years ago, and since then is widely used in medicine as an anticoagulant drug, administered for parenteral, intravenous and subcutaneous. Antithrombin (AT) is a small protein molecule that inactivates several enzymes of the coagulation system. This book discusses the clinical applications of heparin; new antithrombotic and anti-platelet drugs that can be used instead of heparin; and heparin's effect on vascular health.

Chapter I - Heparin catalyzes antithrombin function, especially on IIa and Xa factors. Heparins are divided into two major groups: unfractionated heparin (UH), discovery over 90 years ago and in medical use from the 30s, that is a glycosaminoglycan of great molecular weight (from 3000 to 30000 Dalton); Low molecular weight heparin (LMWH) that are fragments of native heparin, obtained by its chemical or enzymatic depolymerization (molecular weight 4000-5000 Dalton average). Heparin consist of a variably sulphate repeating disaccharide unit. Heparin implements its anticoagulant action by binding to AT through an active molecular fragment: the pentasaccharide sequence.

UH is commonly used during some invasive medical procedures (i.e., hemodialysis). It is also used in primary prevention of venous thromboembolism (VTE) in high risk subjects but in this case LMWH and fondaparinux are more effective, easier in clinical management and equivalent in security. Another field of application of UH is the treatment of VTE though American College of Chest Physicians (ACCP) evidence-based clinical practice guidelines 9th ed. 2012 suggest to use as first option LMWH and Fondaparinux versus UH. Finally, the use of UE is indicated in the early treatment of Non ST-elevation myocardial infarction (N-STEMI) in association with antiplatelet agents . In therapeutic management of ST-elevation myocardial infarction (STEMI) if patient is about to undergoes to primary percutaneous coronary intervention (PCI), UH must be used in patients not receiving bivalirudin or enoxaparin. In fibrinolytic therapy anticoagulation is recommended in STEMI patients treated with lytics until revascularization (if performed) or for the duration of hospital stay up to 8 days, the anticoagulant can be UH as alternative to Enoxaparin, that's the first line anticoagulant. For several years LMWH and fondaparinux have become the treatment of choice for prophylaxis and treatment of VTE. In fact they have a better pharmacokinetics than UH, which allows the routine use in a fixed dose without the need for laboratory controls assays. The dosage is determined by the weight of the patient, kidney function and the specific therapeutic indication.

Chapter II – Acute cardiovascular indications have been treated using heparin therapy for more than 50 years, and it remains widely used today. Unfractionated heparin was a serendipitous find by Jay McLean in 1916 and was traditionally used as a prophylactic measure in surgical thrombosis. Heparin owes its potent anticoagulant activity to antithrombin (AT), a natural inhibitor in the blood. The heparin-AT complex results in the catalytic inhibition of serine proteases in the coagulation cascade, ultimately preventing clot formation. The limitations of heparin have come to the fore through its widespread and long-standing use, with the result that pharmaceutical companies have embarked on the development of more predictable antagonists of clotting.

The action of heparin and its inability for oral administration means that it can only be administered in the hospital setting. New anticoagulants coming online include both parenteral and oral inhibitors. Enhanced selectivity and specificity are also important features of these new anticoagulants, with drugs targeting specific steps in the coagulation cascade such as thrombin or factor Xa. As a result, it is suggested that less laboratory monitoring is needed owing to their more predictable response profiles. However, new clinical guidelines suggest a more cautious approach where certain patient cohorts are concerned.

This chapter will review the story of heparin and its evolution, while exploring the new era of anticoagulant therapy. It will look at the range of drugs currently used in clinical practice, as well as newer drugs that are being developed and are currently in clinical trials, a brief look at anti-platelet therapy, as well as looking at the impact that some of these drugs are having on the prevention and treatment of thromboembolic disease.

Chapter III – Heparin is a highly negatively charged heterogeneous compound, derived from animal tissue that has been used as an antithrombotic drug for more than 70 years. It is generally believed that the efficacy of heparin as an antithrombotic agent is primarily due to its anticoagulant mechanism where it acts to catalyze antithrombin III and heparin cofactor II, natural inhibitors of activated coagulation factors. However, because of its negative charge, administered heparins bind to many cationic molecules present in the circulation and on the vessel wall, particularly the endothelium. There is considerable evidence that the interaction of heparins with the vessel wall not only contributes to the antithrombotic effects of heparins but may be important in preventing vascular disorders thus contributing to vascular health. There is evidence that the interaction of heparin and heparin-like compounds with the vasculature, may be of benefit in the prevention and treatment of atherosclerosis and its complications. The continued successful application of heparin in the design and engineering of stents used for the treatment of atherosclerosis underlines the important role that this drug plays in the health of the vessel wall. Thus the interaction of heparin and related compounds with the blood vessels may contribute to vascular health and have benefits that require further exploration and development.

Chapter IV – Heparin-binding epidermal growth factor (EGF)-like growth factor (HB-EGF), a heparin-interacting protein, is synthesized as a type I transmembrane protein (proHB-EGF) in the ER, transported through the exocytic pathway, and expressed on the cell surface. Subsequently, proHB-EGF or a cleaved form, the carboxyl-terminal fragment of HB-EGF (HB-EGF-CTF), undergoes endocytosis and retrograde transport to several intracellular destinations including the Golgi, ER, lysosome, and inner nuclear membrane (INM). Because they are internalized by endocytosis, cell-surface receptors and ligands can be used for drug delivery. At steady state, most endocytosed proteins are returned to the plasma membrane via endosomal recycling pathways; proteins that are not recycled are transported to distinct destinations. Well-defined membranes surround organelles, emphasizing the significance of the transport pathways that lead to distinct destinations. Thus, the choice of appropriate targets that are promptly transported to specific intracellular compartments is crucial for drug delivery. Here, the author describes the intracellular transport of HB-EGF, focusing on retrograde transport pathways, and discuss the possibilities for exploiting HB-EGF transport in future drug-delivery systems.

In: Heparin
Editor: Nicole B. Wilkinson

ISBN: 978-1-63117-624-1

Chapter I

Heparin: Which Molecule? What Clinical Applications?

Egidio Imbalzano*[1,*], *M.D.*, *Michele Creazzo*[1], *M.D.*, *Giovanni Trapani*[1], *M.D.*, *Antonio Stellitano*[1], *M.D.*, *Marta Zucco*[2], *M.D.*, *Sebastiano Quartuccio*[1], *M.D.*, *Giuseppina Lizio*[1], *Giuseppe Dattilo*[2], *M.D.* and *Antonino Saitta*[1], *M.D.

[1]Department of Internal Medicine, University of Messina, Italy
[2]Department of Cardiology, University of Messina, Italy

Abstract

Heparin is a highly sulphated glycosaminoglycan discovered about 90 years ago, and since then widely used in Medicine as an anticoagulant drug, administered for parenteral, intravenous and subcutaneous. Antithrombin (AT) is a small protein molecule that inactivates several enzymes of the coagulation system. Heparin catalyzes antithrombin function, especially on IIa and Xa factors.

* Corresponding author: Egidio Imbalzano, M.D. Unità Operativa Complessa di Medicina Interna, Azienda Ospedaliera Universitaria "Policlinico G. Martino", Via Consolare Valeria n.1, 98125 Messina, Italy. E-mail: eimbalzano@unime.it. Phone: +393392894665.

Heparins are divided into two major groups: unfractionated heparin (UH), discovery over 90 years ago and in medical use from the 30s, that is a glycosaminoglycan of great molecular weight (from 3000 to 30000 Dalton); Low molecular weight heparin (LMWH) that are fragments of native heparin, obtained by its chemical or enzymatic depolymerization (molecular weight 4000-5000 Dalton average). Heparin consist of a variably sulphate repeating disaccharide unit. Heparin implements its anticoagulant action by binding to AT through an active molecular fragment: the pentasaccharide sequence.

UH is commonly used during some invasive medical procedures (ex. hemodialysis). It is also used in primary prevention of venous thromboembolism (VTE) in high risk subjects but in this case LMWH and fondaparinux are more effective, easier in clinical management and equivalent in security. Another field of application of UH is the treatment of VTE though American College of Chest Physicians (ACCP) evidence-based clinical practice guidelines 9th ed. 2012 suggest to use as first option LMWH and Fondaparinux versus UH. Finally, the use of UE is indicated in the early treatment of Non ST-elevation myocardial infarction (N-STEMI) in association with antiplatelet agents. In therapeutic management of ST-elevation myocardial infarction (STEMI) if patient is about to undergoes to primary percutaneous coronary intervention (PCI) , UH must be used in patients not receiving bivalirudin or enoxaparin. In fibrinolytic therapy anticoagulation is recommended in STEMI patients treated with lytics until revascularization (if performed) or for the duration of hospital stay up to 8 days, the anticoagulant can be UH as alternative to Enoxaparin, that's the first line anticoagulant. For several years LMWH and fondaparinux have become the treatment of choice for prophylaxis and treatment of VTE. In fact they have a better pharmacokinetics than UH, which allows the routine use in a fixed dose without the need for laboratory controls assays. The dosage is determined by the weight of the patient, kidney function and the specific therapeutic indication.

Heparin (H.) is a highly sulphated glycosaminoglycan discovered about 90 years ago, and since then widely used in Medicine as an anticoagulant drug, administered for parenteral, intravenous and subcutaneous. Antithrombin (AT) is a small protein molecule that inactivates several enzymes of the coagulation system. H. catalyzes antithrombin function, especially on IIa and Xa factors. Heparins are divided into two major groups: unfractionated heparin (UFH), discovery over 90 years ago and in medical use from the 30s, that is a glycosaminoglycan of great molecular weight (from 3000 to 30000 Dalton); Low molecular weight heparins (LMWH's) that are fragments of native h., obtained by its chemical or enzymatic depolymerization (molecular weight 4000-5000 Dalton average). They have entered the market since the early 90's and since then their use in daily clinical practice has grown gradually. Compared to UFH, LMWH's have same advantages: no need to monitoring coagulation parameter; smaller risk of bleeding, of osteoporosis in long-term use and of heparin induced thrombocytopenia (HIT), potential side effect. H. consists of a variably sulphate repeating disaccharide unit and implements its anticoagulant action by binding to AT through an active molecular fragment: the pentasaccharide sequence [1, 2].

Unfractionated Heparin

UFH is commonly used during some invasive medical procedures (ex. hemodialysis). It is also used in primary prevention of venous thromboembolism (VTE) in high risk subjects but in this case LMWH's are more effective, easier in clinical management and equivalent in security. Another field of application of UFH is the treatment of VTE though American College of Chest Physicians (ACCP) evidence-based clinical practice guidelines 9th ed. 2012 suggest to use as first option LMWH's and Fondaparinux versus UFH [3]. Finally, the use of UFE is indicated in the early treatment of Non ST-elevation myocardial infarction (N-STEMI) in association with antiplatelet agents [4]. In therapeutic management of ST-elevation myocardial infarction (STEMI) if patient is about to undergoes to primary percutaneous coronary intervention (PCI), UFH must be used in patients not receiving bivalirudin or enoxaparin. In fibrinolytic therapy, anticoagulation is recommended in STEMI patients treated with lytics until revascularization (if performed) or for the duration of hospital stay up to 8 days, the anticoagulant can be UFH as alternative to Enoxaparin, that's the first line anticoagulant [5]. Protamine sulfate (1 mg for 100 international unit (IU) of heparin given over the past 4 hours) is the antidote for the heparin overdose.

Dalteparin

Dalteparin (D.) was put on market in 1993 [6]. It is constituted by a mixture of polysaccharides derived from fragmentation of heparin extracted from pig intestinal mucosa, with a mean molecular weight of 5000 Dalton. D.

selectively inhibits coagulation factors Xa and XII with slight effect on prothrombin time. The use of the drug is indicated for the prophylaxis of VTE in general and orthopaedic surgery, prophylaxis of clotting in extra-corporeal hemodialysis and hemofiltration up to 4 hours, in the treatment of acute deep vein thrombosis (DVT), unstable angina and Non ST Elevation Myocardial Infarction (STEMI) in association with acetil salicilic acid (ASA).

An important placebo-controlled trial based on acutely ill medical patients (PREVENT n=3706) showed that D. 5000 IU sc. once daily was more effective than placebo to prevent VTE with a relative risk reduction of 45% [7].

PROTECT trial (PROphylaxis for ThromboEmbolism in Critical Care Trial) showed that Dalteparin 5000 IU s.c. once daily wasn't more effective than UFH 5000 IU twice daily in prevention of proximal leg DVT, but pulmonary embolism was significantly lower in the D. group versus UFH group [8].

The overall incidence of haemorrhagic complications observed with D. therapy is no greater than that associated with UFH, and data suggest that perioperative transfusion requirements and frequency of bleeding are lower after D [9].

The FRISC II study showed that in patients with unstable coronary artery disease (UCAD) D. in association with intensive therapeutic strategy (coronary angiography and, if appropriate, revascularization, within 7 days from admission) further improves prognosis of patients treated [10].

A meta regression analysis made in 2012 suggest comparable safety and efficacy between D. and enoxaparin in patient undergoing abdominal surgery and in acutely ill medical patients [11].

Bemiparin

Bemiparin (B.) is LMWH that has been available in Europe for 12 years and is indicated for thromboprophylaxis and the treatment of DTV as well as for the prevention of clotting in the extracorporeal circuit during hemodialysis. It's produced through alkaline degradation of swine mucous membrane's heparin and it's termed a 'second-generation' LMWH, because at 3.6 k Dalton (3- 4,2 kDa), it has a lower mean molecular weight than other LMWH and a narrow distribution of saccharide chain lengths, with most being less than 6 kDa. The percent of saccharide chain with weight between 2000 e 6000 D (with only anti-Xa activity) are 50-70%, meanwhile the percent of saccharide chain with weight more than 6000 D (whit anti-hero activity and then with anticoagulant activity) are less than 15%. So it has low anti factor IIa activity and an anti Xa: anti IIa activity ratio of 8:1 compared with a ratio of 1:1 for unfractioned heparin: this means that bemiparin has a better antithrombotic effect and a less bleeding risk. Bemiparin is rapidly absorbed after subcutaneous administration, attaining maximal plasma anti-Xa activity within 2-6 h.

The bioavailability of bemiparin was estimated at 96% and the apparent volume of distribution was 5.1 L. Plasma anti-Xa activity was maintained for up to 12 h with single bemiparin doses of 2500 IU anti-Xa or less and for up to 20-24 h with single doses of 7500-12,500 IU. Bemiparin has the longest half-life of all LMWH's at 5.3 h compared with 0.5-1.0 h for UFH. Elimination is linear, with a mean residence time of over 7 h and total clearance of 0.9 L/h. B. thus has good antithrombotic activity and a better pharmacological profile than UFH. Surgery in patients whit low-moderate risk of DVT: 2500 UI anti Xa sub cutaneous of B. has to be administer 2 hours before or 6 hours after the intervention, then in the next 7/10 days 2500 UI anti Xa s.c. has to be administer until the risk of DVT is decreased [12]. Different trials have proved the efficacy of B. in the prophylaxis of venous thromboembolism. The B. assessment group [13] demonstrates that B., in a single daily subcutaneous dose of 3,500 anti-Xa IU in high risk patients undergoing hip arthroplasty is more effective than UFH administered twice daily at a dose of 5,000 IU in the prevention of postoperative VTE. Both agents are equally safe. Ferriols-Lisart R et al. [14] have demonstrated that B. seems to be as effective and safe as the other LMWH's in the prevention of thromboembolic complications in orthopaedic surgery. Another trial [15] shows also that B. started postoperatively is as effective and safe as enoxaparin started preoperatively in the prevention of venous thromboembolism in patients undergoing total knee replacement.

In the CANBERSURE study [16] in particular was demonstrated that four weeks compared with 1 week of prophylaxis with B. after abdominal or pelvic cancer surgery did not significantly reduce the primary efficacy outcome, but decreased VTE without increasing haemorrhagic complications. Treatment of DVT: The raccomanded dose of B. in the acute phase of DVT is 115 UI/kg/die sc, according to the weight of the patient (5.000 UI/0,2 ml if weight is < 50 kg; 7.500 UI/0,3 ml for patient of 50-70 kg; 10.000 UI/0,4 ml if the weight is> 70 kg). Kakkar et all [17] have demonstrated that the efficacy in terms of recurrence of venous thromboembolism and safety of B. is similar to UFH. B.

is also an effective alternative to warfarin for long-term treatment. In selected patient [18] B. may be a safer and cost-neutral alternative to Vitamnin K antagonist (VKA) for long-term treatment of DVT. Prevention of clotting in the extracorporeal circuit during hemodialysis: During hemodialysis the dose of B. that prevent clotting in the extracorporeal circuit is 2500 UI for patient with weight inferior to 60 Kg, and of 3500 UI for patient with weight more then 60 Kg. Anyway there are no studies that define the adjustment of the dose of B. in the patient with kidney or hepatic diseases. The side effects most frequently reported with B. is a haematoma at the injection site; in the study of comparison of enoxaparin with B. that event was recorded in 22.7 % of patients treated with B. and 32.5 % of those treated with enoxaparin (p = 0.03). In comparison with enoxaparin, there were no other differences in terms of total bleeding, major bleeding and transfusions [15]. In the study of comparison of B. vs. UFH for prophylaxis in abdominal surgery 3 patients in the UFH group were subjected to transfusion and 2 re- operated for bleeding compared with none in the group B. [14]. The changes in haemoglobin levels were similar in both groups. The frequency of ecchymosis in injection site was significantly higher in the control group vs. the group treated with B. (p = 0.015). In the only study of treatment of DVT, the frequency of major and minor bleeding complications is similar in the 3 groups (UFH + warfarin, warfarin and B. + B. alone) [5]. Mild thrombocytopenia was observed in a similar number of patients (3.2 % and 2.6 % B. enoxaparin prophylaxis in the study , UFH 2.0 % and 1.9 % and 3.2 % B. in the study treatment) and had no sequelae. Among the laboratory parameters was observed an increase in γ-GT in 39.3 % of patients in B. group vs 35.7 % in the enoxaparin group and in 47% of patients receiving B. and in 66% of the UFH group in the study of treatment of DVT [15, 16].

Enoxaparin

Enoxaparin (E.) is obtained from porcine intestinal mucosa, that inhibits reactions that lead to the clotting of blood. It's an acidic mucopolysaccharide formed of equal parts of sulphated D-glucosamine and D-glucuronic acid with sulfaminic bridges. Its molecular weight ranges from 3800 to 5000 dalton (mean molecular weight of approximately 4500 dalton). E. binds to and accelerates the activity of antithrombin III. By activating antithrombin III, E. potentiates the inhibition of coagulation factors Xa (that catalyzes the

conversion of prothrombin to thrombin) and IIa (preventing the conversion of fibrinogen to fibrin). E. also prevents the formation of a stable fibrin clot by inhibiting the activation of the fibrin stabilizing factor. [19].

The absolute bioavailability of E. after subcutaneous injection, based on anti-Xa activity, is close to 100%. The mean maximum plasma anti-Xa activity is observed 3 to 5 hours after subcutaneous injection. Plasma anti-hero activity after subcutaneous administration is approximately ten-fold lower than anti-Xa activity. The mean maximum plasma anti-hero activity is observed approximately 3 to 4 hours following subcutaneous injection. The volume of distribution of E. anti-Xa activity is about 5 litres and is close to the blood volume. E. is a low clearance drug. Elimination appears monophasic with a half-life of about 4 hours after a single-subcutaneous dose to about 7 hours after repeated dosing. E. is primarily metabolised in the liver by desulfation and/or depolymerisation to lower molecular weight species with much reduced biological potency. Renal clearance of active fragments represents about 10% of the administered dose and total renal excretion of active and non-active fragments 40% of the dose [20].

E. is indicated: for prophylaxis of deep vein thrombosis in surgical patients and in medical patients who are at risk for thromboembolic complications due to severely restricted mobility; for treatment of deep vein thrombosis with or without pulmonary embolism; for treatment of unstable angina and non-Q-wave myocardial infarction, administered with aspirin; for treatment of acute ST-segment Elevation Myocardial Infarction (STEMI), including patients to be managed medically or with subsequent Percutaneous Coronary Intervention (PCI); for blood clot prevention during hemodialysis.

Dosage and administration. Prophylaxis of DVT: in patients with a moderate risk of thromboembolism, the recommended E. dosage is 2000 IU anti-Xa (0.2 ml) subcutaneously once daily.

In patients with high risk of thromboembolism and in particular in patients undergoing orthopaedic surgery, the recommended E. dosage is 4000 IU anti-Xa (0.4 ml) subcutaneously once daily. Prophylaxis should be continued once daily for 7 to 10 days or until the risk of thromboembolism has diminished and the patient can begin ambulating.

In medical bedridden patients with high risk of thromboembolism, the recommended dose is 4000 IU once daily by subcutaneous injection. Treatment is prescribed for a minimum of 6 days and continued until the return to full ambulation, for a maximum of 14 days. Treatment of venous thrombosis: the recommended dosage for treatment of established DVT is 100 IU/kg body weight twice daily (every 12 hours) subcutaneously for 10 days.

Treatment of Unstable Angina and Non-Q-Wave Myocardial Infarction: the recommended dose of E. is 100 IU/kg every 12 hours by subcutaneous injection, administered concurrently with oral acetylsalicylic acid (100 to 325 mg once daily). Treatment with E. in these patients should be prescribed for a minimum of 2 days and continued until clinical stabilization. The duration of treatment is usually 2 to 8 days. Treatment of Acute ST-segment Elevation Myocardial Infarction: the recommended dose of E. is a single intravenous bolus of 3000 IU plus a 100 IU/kg subcutaneous dose, followed by 100 IU/kg administered subcutaneously every 12 hours (maximum 10000 IU for each of the first two subcutaneous doses only, followed by 100 IU/kg dosing for the remaining doses). When administered in conjunction with a thrombolytic (fibrin-specific or non-fibrin specific), E. should be given between 15 minutes before and 30 minutes after the start of fibrinolytic therapy. All patients should receive ASA as soon as they are identified as having STEMI (75 to 325 mg once daily, unless contraindicated). The recommended duration of E. treatment is 8 days or until hospital discharge. For patients managed with Percutaneous Coronary Intervention (PCI): If the last E. subcutaneous administration was given less than 8 hours before balloon inflation, no additional dosing is needed, otherwise an intravenous bolus of 30 IU/kg of E. should be administered.

Blood clot prevention during hemodialysis: in patients undergoing repeated sessions of hemodialysis, the prevention of thrombosis in the extracorporeal blood circuit is obtained by injection of a dose of 100 IU/kg into the arterial line of the dialysis circuit at the start of the session. The dose is usually sufficient for a 4 hour hemodialysis session. If fibrin rings are formed, a further dose of 50 to 100 IU/kg should be made, depending on the time before the end of the dialysis. In hemodialysed patients with a high risk of haemorrhage, (in particular, in pre or post-operative dialysed patients) or with a progressive haemorrhagic disorder, the dialysis sessions may be carried out by using a dose of 50 IU/kg (double vascular access) or 75 IU/kg (single vascular access).

E. is contraindicated in case of:

- Allergy to E. or its derivatives including other LMWH's.
- Anamnesis positive for HIT
- Acute bacterial endocarditis (with the exception of mechanical prostheses endocarditis).
- Conditions with a high risk of uncontrolled haemorrhage including major bleeding disorders, focal lesions, haemorrhagic stroke, active

ulcerative conditions showing a tendency to haemorrhage (e.g. peptic ulcer, ulcerative colitis).

- Relative contraindications: administration with ticlopidine, non-steroidal anti-inflammatory drugs (NSAIDs), acetylsalicylic acid, platelet antiaggregants.

Many studies have demonstrated the efficacy and safety of E. in medical and surgical patients, both in orthopaedic and oncological surgery. Among the best-known are the ones listed below.

MEDENOX (MEDical patients with ENOXaparin) [1999] was a double-blind, randomized, placebo-controlled trial undertaken to evaluate the efficacy of 2 dosage regimens of E. (40 versus 20 mg) for prevention of VTE in acutely ill medical patients. The primary outcome was VTE between days 1 and 14. The trial showed a significantly reduced risk of venous thromboembolism at the 40-mg dose, compared with the 20 mg group and the placebo group. Furthermore there was no significant difference in the incidence of VTE between the group that received 20 mg of E. and the placebo group [21].

THE-PRINCE (Thromboembolism-Prevention in Cardiopulmonary Diseases with Enoxaparin) [2003] was a randomized trial undertaken to compare E. (40 mg once daily) with UFH (5000 IU three times daily) for the prevention of venous thromboembolic disease in patients with heart failure (HF) or severe respiratory disease. The primary endpoint was the incidence of thromboembolic events up to one day after the treatment period (10 +/- 2 days). The trial underlined the efficacy and safety of E., showing it was at least as effective as UFH in the prevention of thromboembolic events, with significantly fewer adverse events [22].

ENOXACAN II (ENOXAparin in CANcer) [2002] was a randomized, double-blind trial that demonstrated the benefit of extended prophylaxis for VTE after abdominal surgery for cancer. This trial compared a 1-week regimen of E. (40 mg once daily beginning 10 to 14 hours preoperatively and continuing for 6 to 10 days) with a 4-week regimen (40 mg once daily beginning 10 to 14 hours preoperatively and continuing for 25 to 31 days). The primary efficacy endpoint was DVT and the primary safety endpoint was bleeding during the extended-prophylaxis period. This study reported a statistically significant reduction (from 12% to 4.8%) in the rate of postoperative VTE in association with extended prophylaxis as compared with shorter prophylaxis, with no significant differences between groups in the incidence of major or minor bleeding [23].

STEEPLE (SafeTy and Efficacy of Enoxaparin in Percutaneous Coronary Intervention (PCI) patients, an internationaL randomized Evaluation) [2006] was a randomized open-label trial undertaken to assess the safety of E. as compared with that of UFH in elective PCI. The primary endpoint was the incidence of major and minor bleeding at 48 hours after the index PCI (excluding bypass graft bleeding). The main secondary endpoint was the achievement of therapeutic anticoagulation. A single intravenous bolus of E. 0.5 mg/kg and 0.75 mg/kg compared with intravenous UFH (adjusted for activated clotting time) demonstrated superior safety profile of E. injection. It was associated with reduced major and minor bleeding, with a significant reduction at a dose of 0.5 mg per kg, while the 0.75 mg/kg regimen was non-inferior to UFH (6.5% vs. 8.5%). The incidence of major bleeding was significantly reduced in both E. groups. The study also showed that E. was associated with a major rate of patients achieving target anticoagulation levels compared with UFH. No definitive comparison of efficacy in the prevention of ischemic events was provided by this study [24].

BERQVIST (1996) was a randomized trial performed to determine whether an extended-period treatment with E. was more effective as prophylaxis against VTE after total hip replacement, than E. therapy given only during the hospitalization for surgical intervention. The extended-period regimen contemplated a 40 mg dosage of E. once a day during the hospitalization followed by a thromboprophylaxis out of hospital (for a total duration of 30 days). It was compared with a 40 mg dosage of E. once a day, given only during the hospitalization (on average 10-11 days). The incidence of venous thromboembolic complications was significantly lower in patients undergoing elective hip replacement when prophylaxis with E. was given for a total of one month, rather than only during the hospitalization [25].

ESSENCE (Efficacy and Safety of Subcutaneous Enoxaparin in Non-Q-Wave Coronary Events) [1997] was a double-blind comparison of E. with UFH in patients with angina at rest or non–Q-wave myocardial infarction. Patients received either 100 IU of E. per kg of body weight subcutaneously every 12 hours or continuous intravenous UFH, for a minimum of 48 hours to a maximum of 8 days. All patients received 100 mg to 325 mg of ASA daily too. The primary endpoint was the incidence of recurrent angina, myocardial infarction or death; it was significantly lower in the E. group compared with the UFH group after 14 days and remained significant after 30 days. The need for coronary revascularization procedures at 30 days was also significantly less frequent in the patients assigned to E. Although there was no difference in the incidence of major bleeding complications between the two groups, there was a significantly higher incidence of minor haemorrhagic events in the E. group. The trial demonstrated the superiority of E. administrated with ASA in reducing the incidence of ischemic events [26].

ExTRACT-TIMI 25 (Enoxaparin and Thrombolysis Reperfusion for Acute Myocardial Infarction Treatment) [2006] was a randomized, double-blind study with the primary objective to determine whether E. was superior to UFH as adjunctive therapy in patients with Acute ST-Segment Elevation Myocardial Infarction receiving fibrinolytic therapy . The primary efficacy end point was death or non-fatal recurrent myocardial infarction through 30 days. The trial demonstrated the superiority of E. over UFH in reducing death or non-fatal myocardial, but was associated with an increase in major bleeding episodes [27].

EXCLAIM study (Extended CLinical prophylaxis in Acutely Ill Medical patients) [2007] showed the efficacy and safety of extended-duration thromboprophylaxis using E. 40 mg once daily for 28 +/- 4 days, after the standard regimen of E. (40 mg once daily for 10 +/- 4 days), in acutely ill medical patients with recent reduced mobility. Compared to the standard regimen, the 38 +/- 4 days one demonstrated a significantly reduced incidence of VTE and symptomatic DVT. The incidence of major bleeding episodes was higher during the extended duration prophylaxis phase but the rates of total events were low. There was no difference in terms of mortality between the two groups [28].

Recently, the fixed-dose heparin in the prophylaxis of DVT has been questioned, especially in high-risk and obese patients [29]. A weight-based dosing with enoxaparin in morbidly obese (0,5 mg/kg TD) proved to be sufficient in achieving anti-factor Xa levels within the appropriate prophylactic range (range 0.20 – 0.59 IU/ml) without additional adverse effects [30].

Nadroparin

Nadroparin (N.) had a mean molecular weight of 4.5 kD, composed of a mixture pentasaccharide molecules, which is the specific site for high affinity binding to the plasma protein antithrombin III (ATIII). This binding leads to an accelerated inhibition of factor Xa, which accounts for the majority of the antithrombotic effect of nadroparin [31]. N. has a greater ratio of anti-factor Xa to anti-factor Ha activity, greater bioavailability and a longer duration of action, allowing it to be administered by subcutaneous injection for prophylaxis or treatment of thromboembolic disorders, in general surgery and in orthopaedic surgery, treatment of DVT, treatment of unstable angina and non-Q wave myocardial.

N. compared with UFH, in clinical trials conducted for DVT, was effective as UFH in preventing DVT and PE [32-35].

N. was also at least as effective as enoxaparin or oral acenocoumarol in preventing thromboembolic events following general, orthopaedic and oncologic surgery.

When used as prophylaxis, no significant differences in bleeding complications were noted between N. and UFH or acenocoumarol recipients [36-38]. When used for treatment of established DVT N. was as effective as intravenous UFH [39-40]. Subcutaneous N., at dosages similar to those used for the treatment of DVT, in older patients with pulmonary embolism is effective and safe [41].

The FRAX.I.S study, a multi-centre, prospective, randomized, double-blind study show N. provides similar efficacy and safety to treatment with UFH, in the therapeutic management of acute unstable angina or non-Q wave myocardial infarction. [42] N. is well tolerated by older patients. The most frequently reported adverse events in a large (n approximately 4500) placebo-controlled study in general surgical patients were wound and injection site haematoma (11.8 and 10.2%, respectively, vs approximately 6.5% for placebo). When used as treatment for DVT, N. was generally associated with lower occurrences of major bleeding than intravenous UFH (0.5 to 2.3% vs 2 to 5%) [43]. Prophylactic use of N. was associated with significantly fewer adverse events than enoxaparin in high-risk general surgery patients [38].

Parnaparin

Parnaparin (P.) is available in medicine from 1993, and is indicated in DVT prophylaxis in general and orthopaedic surgery for patients at increased risk and in treatment of DVT. P. was at least as effective as UFH in preventing DVT across all clinical trials; and in two large studies in patients undergoing general surgery (n = 610, and n = 173, respectively) the incidence of DVT in the parnaparin (3200 or 6400 IUaXa once-daily) group was statistically significantly lower than in the UFH (5000 IU 2- or 3-times daily) group (3.2% vs 6.3%, P <0.05; and 1.1% vs 7.1%, P = 0.038, respectively). In all studies conducted to test the efficacy in the treatment of DVT parnaparin was at least as effective as the comparator (UFH and nadroparin) in preventing recurrent extending DVT and PE, with a similar safety profile [44]. The PRIME CARE study (a prospective and multi-centre trial 897 adult patients of both sexes suffering from unstable angina), demonstrated that P., in addition to the standard treatment of unstable angina, reduced the incidence of combined triple end points of death, myocardial infarction and need for revascularization when compared to UFH. This benefit was observed at 7 days as well as at 30 days of follow-up. The incidence of minor bleeding was significantly less in patients treated with P. Thus, once daily administration of P. 6400 IU as a fixed dose is a safe and effective alternative to UFH in the treatment of unstable angina [45].

Heparin might possess anti-thrombotic properties other than anticoagulation. The process of depolymerization of heparin to obtain parnaparin resulted in an increased, anticoagulant-independent effect on platelet-polymorphonuclear leukocyte function. Thus, the overall anti-thrombotic properties of parnaparin may be partly due to a leukocyte-mediated anti-inflammatory effect [46]. STEFLUX (Superficial ThromboEmbolism and Fluxum on 664 patients) study was made to investigate the role and the optimal dose and duration of parnaparin in treatment of lower limb superficial vein thrombosis (SVT). The result was that an intermediate dose of P. (8500 IU o.d. for 10 days followed by 6400 IU o.d. for 20 days) was superior to either a 30-day prophylactic dose (4250 IU o.d.) or a 10-day intermediate dose (8500 IU o.d. for 10 days followed by placebo 20 days). No major haemorrhages occurred [47].

Reviparin

Reviparin (R.) has been in use in medical practice since 1994 and it's a second generation LMWH. R. is obtained from porcine intestinal mucosa and is indicated to prevent DVT in general and orthopaedic patients at high risk, in treatment of DVT with or without PE, prevention of acute events in percutaneous transluminal coronary angioplasty (PTCA). R. has been shown to be as effective as UFH in thromboprophylaxis and it has less incidence of local haematoma at injection site. It was found to be as effective as UFH in preventing DVT in moderate risk surgery (general and abdominal) and reducing to a significant extent DVT in patients with brace immobilisation of the legs. In patients with acute VTE, R. was more effective than UFH in thrombus reduction and at least as effective as UFH in the prevention of clinical recurrence of DVT and/or PE, with a similar or lower incidence of bleeding complication than UFH [48-49]. The results of CREATE trial (Clinical trial of Reviparin and Metabolic Modulation in Acute Myocardial Infarction Treatment Evaluation) suggested that R. reduces mortality and re-infarction without a substantive increase in overall stroke in patients with acute ST-segment elevation or new left bundle-branch block myocardial infarction (MI) [50].

For several years LMWHs have become the treatment of choice for prophylaxis and treatment of VTE and in acute coronary diseases. They have a better pharmacokinetics than UH, which allows the routine use in a fixed dose without the need for laboratory controls assays. The dosage is determined by the weight of the patient, kidney function and the specific therapeutic indication.

The big family of anticoagulants is constantly expanding. LMWH's, with their discovery in the medical field, revolutionized the daily management of anticoagulation therapy.

New anticoagulant drugs, for some years in use, can make a new revolution in this field of medicine. Fondaparinux, synthetic pentasaccharide factor Xa inhibitor, has given great results and important new hopes for the future. Direct Thrombin Inhibitors exert their antithrombotic effect through direct, selective, and reversible binding to the active site of thrombin. Dabigatran, rivaroxaban, and apixaban are novel oral anticoagulants that offer major advantages over current agents. They have rapid onset and more predictable anticoagulants response that eliminates the need for monitoring [51].

References

[1] Cox M, Nelson D. 2004, Lehninger, *Principles of Biochemistry,* Freeman, p. 1100.

[2] Eikelboom JW, Hankey GJ, Low molecular weight heparins and heparinoids, *Med. J. Aust.* 2002 Oct 7; 177 (7):379-83.

[3] Yngve Falck-Ytter, Charles W. Francis, Norman A. Johanson ,Catherine Curley , Ola E. Dahl et al. Prevention of VTE in Orthopedic Surgery Patients: Antithrombotic Therapy and Prevention of Thrombosis, 9th ed:

American College of Chest Physicians Evidence-Based Clinical Practice Guidelines Yngve Falck-Ytter, MD et al. *Chest* 2012;141(2_suppl): e278S-e325S. doi:10.1378/chest.11-2404.

[4] Hamm CW et al. ESC Guidelines for the management of acute coronary syndromes in patients presenting without persistent ST-segment elevation. *European Heart Journal* 2011, 32, 2999-3054. doi 10.1093/ eurheartj/ehr236.

[5] Steg PG et al, Guidelines for the management of acute myocardial infarction in patients presenting with ST-segment elevation. *European Heart Journal* 2012, 33, 2569-2619. doi 10.1093/eurheartj/ehr215

[6] Howard PA Dalteparin: a low-molecular-weight heparin. *Ann. Pharmacother.* 1997 Feb;31(2):192-203.

[7] Leizorovicz A, Cohen AT, Turpie AG, Olsson CG, Vaitkus PT, Goldhaber SZ, PREVENT Medical Thromboprophylaxis Study Group. Randomized, placebo-controlled trial of dalteparin for the prevention of venous thromboembolism in acutely ill medical patients. *Circulation* 2004 Aug 17; 110(7):874-9. Epub 2004 Aug 2.

[8] Cook D et al. Dalteparin versus unfractionated heparin in critically ill patients. PROTECT investigators for the Canadian Clinical care Trials Groups and the Australian and New Zealand Intensive Care Society Clinical Trials Group. *N. Engl. J. Med.* 2011 Apr 7;364(14):1305-14. doi: 10.1056/NEJMoa1014475. Epub 2011 Mar 22.

[9] Dunn CJ, Sorkin EM. Dalteparin sodium. A review of its pharmacology and clinical use in the prevention and treatment of thromboembolic disorders. *Drugs* 1996 Aug; 52(2):276-305.

[10] Lagerqvist B, Husted S, Kontny F, Ståhle E, Swahn E, Wallentin L 5-year outcomes in the FRISC II randomised trial of an invasive versus a non-invasive strategy in non-ST-elevation acute coronary syndrome: a follow-up study. Fast Revascularisation during InStability in Coronary artery disease (FRISC II) Investigators. *Lancet.* 2006 Sep 16; 368(9540): 998-1004.

[11] Dranitsaris G, Jelincic V, Choe Y. Meta-regression analysis to indirectly compare prophylaxis with dalteparin or enoxaparin in patients at high risk for venous thromboembolic events. *Clin. Appl. Thromb. Hemost.* 2012 Jun; 18(3):233-42. Doi: 10.1177/1076029611426869. Epub 2012 Mar 2. Review.

[12] Sanchez-Ferrer CF Bemiparin: pharmacologocal profile. *Drugs* 2010 dec 14;70 suppl 2:19-23 doi 10.2165/1158581.

[13] Kakkar VV, Howes J, Sharma V, Kadziola Z. A comparative double-blind, randomised trial of a new second generation LMWH (bemiparin) and UFH in the prevention of post-operative venous thromboembolism. The Bemiparin Assessment group. *J. Thromb. Haemost.* 2000 Apr.; 83(4): 523-9.
[14] Ferriols-Lisart R, Ferriols-Lisart F, Jiménez-Torres V. Effectiveness and safety of bemiparin versus low-molecular weight heparins in orthopaedic surgery. *Pharm. World Sci.* 2002 Jun; 24(3):87-94.
[15] Navarro-Quilis A, Castellet E, Rocha E, Paz-Jiménez J, Planès A; Efficacy and safety of bemiparin compared with enoxaparin in the prevention of venous thromboembolism after total knee arthroplasty: a randomized, double-blind clinical trial. *J. Thromb. Haemost.* 2003 Mar; 1(3):425-32.
[16] Kakkar VV, Balibrea JL, Martínez-González J, Prandoni P; Extended prophylaxis with bemiparin for the prevention of venous thromboembolism after abdominal or pelvic surgery for cancer: the CANBESURE randomized study. *J. Thromb. Haemost.* 2010 Jun; 8(6): 1223-9. doi: 10.1111/j.1538-7836.2010.03892.x. Epub 2010 Apr 30.
[17] Kakkar VV, Gebska M, Kadziola Z, Saba N, Carrasco P; Low-molecular-weight heparin in the acute and long-term treatment of deep vein thrombosis. *Thromb. Haemost.* 2003 Apr; 89(4):674-80.
[18] Santamaría A, Juárez S, Reche A, Gómez-Outes A, Martínez-González J, Low-molecular-weight heparin, bemiparin, in the outpatient treatment and secondary prophylaxis of venous thromboembolism in standard clinical practice: the ESFERA Study. *Int. J. Clin. Pract.* 2006 May; 60(5): 518-25.
[19] Drugbank CA database.
[20] Clexane ® data sheet.
[21] Turpie AG. Thrombosis prophylaxis in the acutely ill medical patient: insights from the prophylaxis in MEDical patients with ENOXaparin (MEDENOX) trial. *Am. J. Cardiol.* 2000 Dec 28; 86(12B):48M-52M.
[22] Kleber FX, Witt C, Vogel G, Koppenhagen K, Schomaker U, Flosbach CW; THE-PRINCE Study Group. Randomized comparison of enoxaparin with unfractionated heparin for the prevention of venous thromboembolism in medical patients with heart failure or severe respiratory disease. *Am. Heart J.* 2003 Apr; 145(4):614-21.
[23] Bergqvist D, Agnelli G, Cohen AT, Eldor A, Nilsson PE, Le Moigne-Amrani A, Dietrich-Neto F; , for the ENOXACAN II Investigators.

Duration of prophylaxis against venous thromboembolism with enoxaparin after surgery for cancer. *N. Engl. J. Med.* 2002; 346:975-980.

[24] Gilles Montalescot M.D. et al. STEEPLE Investigators. Enoxaparin versus Unfractionated Heparin in Elective Percutaneous Coronary Intervention. *N. Engl. J. Med.* 2006; 355:1006-17.

[25] Bergqvist D, Benoni G, Bjrgell O, Fredin H, Hedlundh U, Nicolas S, Nilsson P, Nylander G. Low-molecular-weight heparin (enoxaparin) as prophylaxis against venous thromboembolism after total hip replacement.. *N. Engl. J. Med.* 1996; 335:696-700.

[26] Cohen M, Demers C, Gurfinkel EP, Turpie AG, Fromell GJ, Goodman S, Langer A, Califf RM, Fox KA, Premmereur J, Bigonzi F. A comparison of low-molecular-weight heparin with unfractionated heparin for unstable coronary artery disease. Efficacy and Safety of Subcutaneous Enoxaparin in Non-Q-Wave Coronary Events Study Group. *N. Engl. J. Med.* 1997 Aug 14; 337(7):447-52.

[27] Antman EM, Morrow DA, McCabe CH, Murphy SA, Ruda M, Sadowski Z, Budaj A, López-Sendón JL, Guneri S, Jiang F, White HD, Fox KA, Braunwald E; ExTRACT-TIMI 25 Investigators. Enoxaparin versus unfractionated heparin with fibrinolysis for ST-elevation myocardial infarction. *N. Engl. J. Med.* 2006 Apr 6; 354(14):1477-88.

[28] Hull RD, Schellong SM, Tapson VF, Monreal M, Samama MM, Nicol P, Vicaut E, Turpie AG, Yusen RD; Extended-duration venous thromboembolism prophylaxis in acutely ill medical patients with recently reduced mobility: a randomized trial. EXCLAIM (Extended Prophylaxis for Venous ThromboEmbolism in Acutely Ill Medical Patients With Prolonged Immobilization) study. *Ann. Intern. Med.* 2010 Jul 6; 153(1):8-18. doi: 10.7326/0003-4819-153-1-201007060-00004.

[29] Imbalzano E, Creazzo M, Mandraffino G, Sardo MA, Saitta A. Treatment failure of low molecular weight heparin in post-surgery orthopedic case. *Int. J. Cardiol.* 2013 Nov 5; 169(3): e36-7. doi: 10.1016/ j.ijcard.2013.08.109.

[30] Ludwig KP, Simons HJ, Mone M, Barton RG, Kimball EJ. Implementation of an enoxaparin protocol for venous thromboembolism prophylaxis in obese surgical intensive care unit patients. *Ann. Pharmacother.* 2011; 45:1356–1362.

[31] Barradell LB, Buckley MM.Nadroparin calcium. A review of its pharmacology and clinical applications in the prevention and treatment of thromboembolic disorders. *Drugs.* 1992 Nov; 44(5):858-88.

[32] Marassi A, Balzano G, Mari G, D'Angelo SV, Della Valle P, Di Carlo V, D'Angelo A Prevention of postoperative deep vein thrombosis in cancer patients. A randomized trial with low molecular weight heparin (CY 216). *Int. Surg.* 1993; 78:166-70.

[33] Kakkar VV, Murray WJ. Efficacy and safety of low-molecular-weight heparin (CY216) in preventing postoperative venous thrombo-embolism: a co-operative study.. *Br. J. Surg.* 1985; 72:786-91.

[34] Comparison of a low molecular weight heparin and unfractionated heparin for the prevention of deep vein thrombosis in patients undergoing abdominal surgery. The European Fraxiparin Study (EFS) Group.. *Br. J. Surg.* 1988; 75:1058-63.

[35] BalasPEet al. Efficacy and safety of nadroparin (Fraxiparine) versus placebo in the prophylactic treatment of deep vein thrombosis in patients with high thrombo-embolic risk undergoing general surgery.01 *Thromb. Res.* 1992; 65(Suppl 1): S113.

[36] Lopaciuk S, Bielska-Falda H, Noszczyk W, Bielawiec M, Witkiewicz W, Filipecki S, Michalak J, Ciesielski L, Mackiewicz Z, Czestochowska E, Zawilska K, Cencora A. Low molecular weight heparin versus acenocoumarol in the secondary prophylaxis of deep vein thrombosis.. *Thromb. Haemost.* 1999;81:26-3.

[37] López-Beret P, Orgaz A, Fontcuberta J, Doblas M, Martinez A, Lozano G, Romero A. Low molecular weight heparin versus oral anticoagulants in the long-term treatment of deep venous thrombosis.. *J. Vasc. Surg.* 2001; 33:77-90.

[38] Simonneau G, Laporte S, Mismetti P, Derlon A, Samii K, Samama CM, Bergman JF. A randomized study comparing the efficacy and safety of nadroparin 2850 IU (0.3 mL) vs. enoxaparin 4000 IU (40 mg) in the prevention of venous thromboembolism after colorectal surgery for cancer.. *J. Thromb. Haemost.* 2006; 4:1693-700.

[39] A randomised trial of subcutaneous low molecular weight heparin (CY 216) compared with intravenous unfractionated heparin in the treatment of deep vein thrombosis. A collaborative European multicentre study.. *Thromb. Haemost.* 1991 Mar 4; 65:251-6.

[40] Prandoni P, Lensing AW, Buller HR, Carta M, Cogo A, Vigo M, Casara D, Ruol A, ten Cate JW. Comparison of subcutaneous low-molecular-weight heparin with intravenous standard heparin in proximal deep-vein thrombosis.. *Lancet* 1992 Feb 22;339:441-5.

[41] Théry C, Simonneau G, Meyer G, Hélénon O, Bridey F, Armagnac C, d'Azemar P, Coquart JP. Randomized trial of subcutaneous low-

molecular-weight heparin CY 216 (Fraxiparine) compared with intravenous unfractionated heparin in the curative treatment of submassive pulmonary embolism. A dose-ranging study.. *Circulation* 1992; 85:1380-9.

[42] Comparison of two treatment durations (6 days and 14 days) of a low molecular weight heparin with a 6-day treatment of unfractionated heparin in the initial management of unstable angina or non-Q wave myocardial infarction: FRAX.I.S. (FRAxiparine in Ischaemic Syndrome). *Eur. Heart J.* 1999;20:1553-62.

[43] Davis R, Faulds D. Nadroparin calcium. A review of its pharmacology and clinical use in the prevention and treatment of thromboembolic disorders. *Drugs Aging* 1997; 10(4):299-322.

[44] Camporese G, Bernardi E, Noventa F. Update on the clinical use of the low molecular weight heparin, parnaparin. *Vasc. Health Risk Manag.* 2009; 5: 819–831. Published online 2009 October 12.

[45] Prime Care Study Investigators Group. Comparative efficacy of once daily parnaparin and unfractionated heparin in unstable angina pectoris: PRIME CARE study. *Indian Heart J.* 2005;57:648–54.

[46] Maugeri N, De Gaetano G, Barbanti M, et al. Prevention of platelet-polymorphonuclear leukocyte interactions: new clues to the antithrombotic properties of parnaparin, a low molecular weight heparin. *Haematologica.* 2005; 90:833–9.

[47] Cosmi B, Filippini M, Tonti D, Avruscio G, Ghirarduzzi A, Bucherini E, Camporese G, Imberti D, Palareti G; STEFLUX Investigators. A randomized double-blind study of low-molecular-weight heparin (parnaparin) for superficial vein thrombosis: STEFLUX (Superficial ThromboEmbolism and Fluxum). *J. Thromb. Haemost.* 2012 Jun; 10(6): 1026-35. doi: 10.1111/j.1538-7836.2012.04727.x.

[48] Gore M, Kelkar P, Rege N, Ross C. Reviparin sodium clivarine, a review of its therapeutic use *J. Indian Med. Assoc.* 2004 Oct; 102(10): 589-90, 592. Review.

[49] Michael R. Lassen, M.D., Lars C. Borris, M.D., and Roumen L. Nakov, M.D., Ph.D. Use of the Low-Molecular-Weight Heparin Reviparin to Prevent Deep-Vein Thrombosis after Leg Injury Requiring Immobilization *N. Eng. J. of Medicine* 2002 347: 726-730. DOI: 10.1056/NEJMoa011327.

[50] Yusuf S, Mehta SR, Xie C, Ahmed RJ, Xavier D, Pais P, Zhu J, Liu L; CREATE Trial Group Investigators. Effects of reviparin, a low-molecular-weight heparin, on mortality, reinfarction, and strokes in

patients with acute myocardial infarction presenting with ST-segment elevation. *JAMA*. 2005 Jan 26; 293(4):427-35.

[51] Alquwaizani M, Buckley L, Adams C, Fanikos J. Anticoagulants: a review of pharmacology, dosing and complications. *Curr. Emerg. Hosp. Med. Resp*. 2013 Apr 21; 1(2): 83-97. Print 2013 Jun.

In: Heparin
Editor: Nicole B. Wilkinson
ISBN: 978-1-63117-624-1

Chapter II

Moving Away from Heparin: The New Antithrombotic and Anti-Platelet Drugs

Leanne F. Harris[1] and Anthony J. Killard[2,3,*]
[1]Biomedical Diagnostics Institute,
National Centre for Sensor Research,
Dublin City University, Dublin, Ireland
[2]Department of Applied Sciences,
University of the West of England, Coldharbour Lane, UK
[3]College of Sciences and Health,
School of Biological Sciences,
Dublin institute of Technology, Dublin, Ireland

Abstract

Acute cardiovascular indications have been treated using heparin therapy for more than 50 years, and it remains widely used today. Unfractionated heparin was a serendipitous find by Jay McLean in 1916 and was traditionally used as a prophylactic measure in surgical

---

* Corresponding Author: Prof. Anthony J. Killard. Department of Applied Sciences, University of the West of England, Coldharbour Lane, Bristol BS16 1QY, UK. Tel: + 00 44 1173282967, Fax: + 00 44 1173282904. E-mail: tony.killard@uwe.ac.uk.

thrombosis. Heparin owes its potent anticoagulant activity to antithrombin (AT), a natural inhibitor in the blood. The heparin-AT complex results in the catalytic inhibition of serine proteases in the coagulation cascade, ultimately preventing clot formation. The limitations of heparin have come to the fore through its widespread and long-standing use, with the result that pharmaceutical companies have embarked on the development of more predictable antagonists of clotting.

The action of heparin and its inability for oral administration means that it can only be administered in the hospital setting. New anticoagulants coming online include both parenteral and oral inhibitors. Enhanced selectivity and specificity are also important features of these new anticoagulants, with drugs targeting specific steps in the coagulation cascade such as thrombin or factor Xa. As a result, it is suggested that less laboratory monitoring is needed owing to their more predictable response profiles. However, new clinical guidelines suggest a more cautious approach where certain patient cohorts are concerned.

This chapter will review the story of heparin and its evolution, while exploring the new era of anticoagulant therapy. It will look at the range of drugs currently used in clinical practice, as well as newer drugs that are being developed and are currently in clinical trials, a brief look at anti-platelet therapy, as well as looking at the impact that some of these drugs are having on the prevention and treatment of thromboembolic disease.

Introduction

Cardiovascular disease is a significant cause of global morbidity and mortality, with thromboembolic diseases remaining a serious problem when it comes to public health [1]. Thromboembolism can arise as a result of both acquired and inherited risk factors and usually ensues when a blood vessel (a veins or artery) becomes obstructed by a clot [2]. Venous thromboembolism (VTE) stands as the third most commonly occurring cardiovascular disease after myocardial infarction and stroke [3]. Anticoagulants or antithrombotics are administered for the prevention and treatment of blood clotting disorders such as VTE [4]. Patients have access to a range of anticoagulant drugs including traditional drugs such as warfarin and heparin, but also newer more specific drugs such as direct and indirect thrombin inhibitors, FXa inhibitors and anti-platelets. While traditional inhibitors of clotting are used routinely in clinical practice, they suffer from many limitations and drawbacks, a problem which has been targeted by major pharmaceutical companies as they endeavour to improve upon and develop more effective antithrombotics [5].

Heparins were discovered almost 100 years ago and have since been used extensively as antithrombotic drugs [6]. While heparin has served its purpose as a potent antithrombotic, it has also set the scene for further advances in drug development. The anticoagulant role of heparin is to bind AT. However, heparin is additionally capable of non-specific binding to other molecules [7]. This non-specific binding can contribute to the inconsistency in responses observed between patients. To account for this increased variability, individuals on UFH therapy need to be monitored regularly. Another drawback of heparin is that it is administered parenterally as it cannot be absorbed orally. Low molecular weight heparins are shorter in chain length than UFHs, at about one third their molecular weight [8]. While LMWHs require less clinical monitoring as a result of their shorter chain lengths and improved pharmacokinetic profiles, they still require administration as injectable drugs. Such limitations have encouraged pharmaceutical companies to focus on the development of new anticoagulants that focus on enhanced selectivity, specificity and oral administration. The first step was the development of LMWH from UFH, followed by the ultra-LMWHs with much shorter chain lengths, factor Xa inhibitors and thrombin inhibitors. This chapter will review the historical perspective of heparin and its low molecular weight counterparts, while also looking at specific clotting factor inhibitors, anti-platelet therapies and the novel antithrombotic drugs that have been, and continue to be, developed.

Heparin

Heparins belong to a group of natural glycosaminoglycans (GAGs) produced in mast cells, and are a heterogeneous mixture of unbranched polysaccharides, including heparan, dermatan, chondroitin, and keratan sulfates [8]. Heparins are extracted and purified from animal tissues, typically of bovine, ovine or porcine origin. With molecular weights ranging from 3,000-15,000 Da in size, the clearance of small and large heparin chains varies, resulting in complex pharmacokinetics [7]. Heparin has the ability to inhibit thrombin, FXa, FX, IXa, XIa and XIIa, with greatest inhibition of thrombin and FXa. It requires AT to exert its anticoagulant effect. AT is a slow endogenous inhibitor of thrombin present in the blood However, once it comes into contact with heparin, a conformational change at its reactive centre allows it to begin the rapid inhibition of both thrombin and FXa [8]. Just one third of the heparin molecule can bind to AT and this specific region has a unique pentasaccharide structure which is referred to as the AT binding domain [9]. While heparin binds AT, it can also non-specifically bind to plasma proteins, platelets, macrophages, and endothelial cells [7]. This binding can often result in reduced anticoagulant activity and decreased therapeutic predictability. As a result, unfractionated heparins require regular monitoring and laboratory testing, which is carried out using the activated partial thromboplastin time test (aPTT).

The clearance of heparin is also related to the chain length of the molecule with high molecular weight molecules being cleared more rapidly than those of lower molecular weights. Clearance is dose-dependent with initial rapid clearance being following by a more gradual rate of clearance. Low doses of heparin are cleared rapidly though a saturable phase followed by a slow, nonsaturable mechanism of clearance which is predominantly renal [8]. UFH has a half-life of 30 minutes once administered subcutaneously or intravenously [8]. This rapid clearance is another disadvantage as it means that without continuous IV feed, the patient is either often under- or over-medicated, with the associated risks of bleeding and clotting.

Other side effects of UFH include heparin induced thrombocytopenia (HIT), an immune-mediated disorder, through the binding of platelet factor 4 (PF4) to heparin which causes a reduction in platelet numbers in the blood [10]. This can either come in the form of a less severe and temporary form in some 10 to 20% of patients (HIT type 1), but in a small number of cases, about 1-3% of patients, it can result in the more serious HIT Type 2. HIT type 1 is a non-immunologic response to heparin which results in platelet clumping within 48-72 hours of heparin administration. HIT type 2 is immune-mediated and is associated with a risk of thrombosis [11]. Heparin is also known to affect bone metabolism resulting in heparin induced osteoporosis with a reduction in bone mineral density [8]. As a result of these HIT related complications in addition to the previously mentioned disadvantages of UFH, it has been largely replaced by safer and more predictable LMWHs in the clinical setting.

Low Molecular Weight Heparins

First developed in the 1980s and commercially available in the 1990s, the synthesis of LMWHs from UFH marked the beginning of the development of new and improved anticoagulants for patient care [12]. LMWHs are derived from UFH through chemical or enzyme depolymerisation processes, to produce short polysaccharide chains of low molecular weights, usually less than 5000 Da. LMWHs have been proven to be more predictable, more reliable and safer than UFH. The shorter chain length results in a longer half-life of 3-6 hours with a more predictable dose-response, thus requiring less laboratory monitoring [8]. The risks of HIT and heparin induced osteoporosis are also lowered with LMWHs.

LMWHs have a reduced ability to inhibit thrombin due to their smaller polysaccharide chain. For thrombin inhibition, heparin must bind to both thrombin and AT and this ternary complex can only be formed in the presence of heparin with a chain length of 18 saccahride units. The smaller fragments of LMWHs are effective inhibitors of FXa and show less non-specific binding to plasma factors, macrophages and endothelial cells and have approximately 90% bioavailability. The aPTT test is ineffective when measuring the activity of LMWH, as it assays anti-factor IIa activity which is not fully inhibited by LMWHs as a result of their smaller molecular weight. While LMWHs are more predictable, as with any drug, its effects will vary from patient to patient. While normal patient cohorts may respond well on LMWH therapy, there are groups of patients that will always require monitoring. LMWHs are cleared renally, indicating that patients with poor kidney function would require monitoring, as would the elderly, pregnant women, children and those patients who are over- or underweight [13]. LMWHs have a half-life of 3 to 4 hours (sub-cutaneous delivery). The chromogenic anti-Xa assay is the 'gold standard' assay currently used in central diagnostic laboratories for monitoring LMWH therapy [14].

LMWHs come in many forms, and do vary in terms of their biological, chemical and physical properties. However, the main difference is their molecular weight. Some of these include: dalteparin, enoxaparin, tinzaparin, nadroparin, and reviparin (Table 1).

Table 1. Characteristics of a selection of LMWH drugs

LMWH	Brand name	Mean Molecular weight (Da)	Anti-Xa/ anti-IIa ratio	Plasma half-life
Dalteparin	Fragmin®	6,000	2.7	3-5 hours
Enoxaparin	Lovenox®	4,500	3.6	4.5 hours
Tinzaparin	Innohep®	6,500	2.8	3.4 hours
Reviprin	Clivarin®	3,900	≥3.6	3.3 hours
Nadroparin	Fraxiparine®	4,300	3.8	7 hours

Direct Thrombin Inhibitors

Thrombin is a model target for anticoagulant development due to its significant and central role in coagulation. As discussed above, it can be inhibited indirectly through the use of UFH, LMWHs and AT. However, direct inhibition is more efficient. The direct inhibition of thrombin will result in a more predictable dose response profile than indirect inhibition [15]. By targeting specific factors in the coagulation cascade, it is believed that drugs with broader therapeutic ranges can be developed. The first direct thrombin inhibitors (DTIs) became available in 1998 and these could be administered either orally or parenterally [12]. DTIs work on the basis of targeting the specific sites on thrombin responsible for clotting. DTIs tend not to bind to plasma proteins or to PF4, which means that DTI activity is not altered or hindered in the presence of platelet-rich thrombin. Thrombin bound to fibrin or fibrin degradation products are often masked and cannot be inhibited by heparin, conversely DTIs can inhibit thrombin bound to fibrin or thrombin bound to platelets [15]. Injectable DTIs include hirudin, desirudin, bivalirudin, lepirudin, and argatroban, while examples of oral DTIs include melagatran and dabigatran (Table 2).

Table 2. Characteristics of a selection of thrombin inhibitors

DTI	Molecular weight (Da)	Plasma half-life	Primary route of clearance	Route of administration
Hirudin	7000	60 minutes	Kidneys	Parenteral
Lepirudin	6979.5	1 hour	Kidneys	Parenteral
Bivalirudin	1980	25 minutes	Liver & kidneys	Parenteral
Desirudin	6963.52	2-3 hours	Kidneys	Parenteral
Argatroban	527	45 minutes	Liver	Parenteral
Dabigatran	628 (prodrug) 472 (active)	12-14 hours	Kidneys	Oral

Parenteral DTIs

Hirudin is a natural inhibitor of thrombin produced by the medicinal leech *Hirudo medicinalis*. It is a 65 amino acid peptide with a molecular weight of 7 kDa. Therapeutic hirudins are produced using recombinant technologies with *Saccharomyces cerevisiae* and differ slightly in structure to natural hirudins

[16]. Hirudins bind to two sites on thrombin, the active site and exosite 1, and are thus referred to as bivalent DTIs (Figure 1). Hirudins have a half-life of 60 minutes after intravenous injection and 120 minutes after subcutaneous injection [17]. Lepirudin and desirudin are recombinant hirudins, and so their recombinant structure confers a slightly lower affinity for thrombin than natural hirudin. Despite this they are considered the most potent of thrombin inhibitors, binding to both the active site and exosite 1 of thrombin.

As already outlined the DTIs are capable of inhibiting clot-bound thrombin, which is true of hirudin as it can inhibit both free and clot-bound thrombin [18,19].

The major drawbacks highlighted by clinicians, is that hirudin's effectiveness depends upon excellent renal function, which can lead to increased bleeding risk and there is currently no antidote available [16].

Lepirudin is a bivalent inhibitor of thrombin that binds irreversibly and is cleared by the kidneys so it must be monitored in patients with renal impairment. It is also approved as an alternative antithrombotic therapy in HIT [4]. The mechanism of action is such that one molecule of lepirudin will bind to one molecule of thrombin and a rapid response is achieved after intravenous injection with a half-life of 1 hour. With renal impairment, the half-life is extended to 2 hours and very often patients treated with hirudin for more than five days can develop anti-hirudin antibodies which will extend the half-life of the drug [20].

Bivalirudin is a synthetic 20 amino acid analogue of hirudin that specifically inhibits thrombin and is recommended for use in percutaneous coronary intervention (PCI) as a result of its ability to reduce bleeding-related complications [21]. It has a short half-life of 25 minutes and, as a bivalent analogue of hirudin, it binds to both the active site and exosite 1 of thrombin (Figure 1).

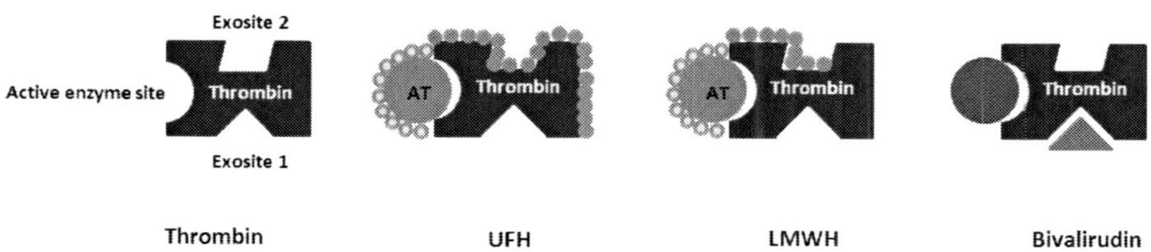

Figure 1. Binding sites of thrombin and interactions with different anticoagulants. (Exosite 1 = fibrin binding site, exosite 2 = heparin binding site).

Inhibition with bivalirudin is reversible and thrombin activity is restored, which ultimately reduces bleeding risk. Its binding to thrombin is transient and it is only partly cleared through the liver and kidneys, reducing bleeding complications but implicating a need for monitoring of patients with renal insufficiency. Owing to its reduced bleeding rates, bivalirudin has been selected as a favoured alternative over UFH and enoxaparin for use in PCI settings and for patients undergoing percutaneous transluminal coronary angioplasty (PTCA) [22].

Argatroban is a low molecular weight (527 Da) DTI and is a synthestic analogue of L-arginine that reversibly binds to the active site on thrombin. It is metabolised and cleared hepatically and as such requires monitoring and subsequent dose adjustment in patients with liver complications but not renal impairment, making it safer for patients with kidney problems [23]. It is licensed in the USA for the prevention and treatment of thrombosis in patients with HIT and can be monitored using aPTT, activated clotting time (ACT) and prothrombin time (PT) assays.

Oral DTIs

The first oral DTI, ximelagatran, the prodrug of melagatran, underwent clinical trials but was withdrawn from the global market in 2006 as a result of concerns posed by the FDA in the USA surrounding possible liver toxicity, with raised alanine transferase activity identified in 6% of subjects. Melagatran was a dipeptide mimetic of Fibrinopeptide A (Fib A) thrombin binding sequence. Modified into a lipophilic prodrug form (ximelagatran), resulting in 20% bioavailability following oral administration. Despite its side effects, it was demonstrated that ximelagatran was as effective as traditional anticoagulants in treating venous and arterial thromboses [23].

Dabigatran (Pradaxa®) inhibits thrombin by binding to its active site via ionic interactions. Dabigatran etexilate is the prodrug that is rapidly converted to dabigatran after absorption. It is a low molecular weight drug that can reversibly bind and inhibit both clot-bound and free thrombin [23]. The hydrophobic prodrug, dabigatran etexilate, prefers to act in an acidic environment and the capsule was designed for release in the stomach, followed by absorption within the small intestine [24]. To minimise the effects of gastric pH on the drug activity, capsules were developed that comprise a core tartaric acid surrounded by dabigatran etexilate, bringing the optimal pH environment to the gastrointestinal tract [25].

Peak plasma concentrations of dabigatran occur within 1.5 to 2 hours after absorption, with a half-life of 9-17 hours, which is dependent upon the age and renal capacity of the patient. The primary route for clearance is through the kidneys and while patients with moderate hepatic impairment require little adjustment of dosage, patients with severe hepatic impairment will require regular monitoring and dose adjustment [23].

Dabigatran has come to the fore as the most promising of DTIs with rapid activity, it does not interact with other drugs or foodstuffs, it has a wide therapeutic range, and an excellent safety record which eliminates the need for routine monitoring [23]. It was approved for use in the USA in 2010 and the UK in 2012 as a replacement for warfarin for the prevention of stroke in patients with atrial fibrillation.

Factor Xa Inhibitors

FXa, as along with thrombin, is another important target in the development of new antithrombotics. FXa occupies a critical position in the coagulation cascade, and can be found at the junction of the extrinsic and intrinsic pathways. It is at this point where FXa acts on prothrombin to convert it to thrombin. Thrombin is the final enzyme in the cascade and is ultimately responsible for converting soluble fibrinogen into an insoluble fibrin clot [26]. FXa inhibitors avoid indirect inhibition such as, vitamin K-dependent clotting factor synthesis as with warfarin, or the activation of AT to inhibit FXa as with heparin or low molecular weight heparin [27].

FXa inhibitors first appeared in 2001 with the development of the very first injectable FXa inhibitor, fondaparinux. This is a chemically formulated sulphated pentasaccharide and it inhibits FXa by reversibly binding to AT [12]. Fondaparinux indirectly, but selectively inhibits FXa and unlike the LMWHs, it does not interfere with thrombin or platelets in its activity and has almost 100% bioavailability. It is cleared renally and must be closely monitored in patients with renal complications but the risk of HIT with fondaparinux is greatly reduced, which is why it is often used as alternative antithrombotic management in HIT [28]. Fondaparinux is also administered for the treatment of deep vein thrombosis and pulmonary embolism and in prophylaxis following hip and knee surgery [4]. Idraparinux is a modification of fondaparinux with higher binding affinity to AT equal to its plasma half-life of 80 to 130 hours. As a result, it had the potential of requiring only weekly dosing. However, phase III trials showed disappointing results in the treatment and management of DVT and AF, with some increased bleeding risks identified [29].

Rivaroxaban was the first example of a direct, oral reversible FXa inhibitor. It is a low molecular weight derivative of oxazolidinone and it is absorbed by the gut and fully active within 4 hours of administration, with a half-life of 8 to 12 hours [30]. Other notable advantages of this inhibitor are its dose proportional pharmacokinetics and low tendency for drug-drug interactions [12], and it requires only daily dosing. When compared with LMWHs, rivaroxaban has shown improved or comparable clinical results for the short-term prevention of VTE and as a prophylactic measure for VTE after orthopaedic surgery, stroke and non-valvular atrial fibrillation [31, 32]. However, it is contraindicated for those with renal or liver dysfunction.

Apixaban is a potent pyrazole-based reversible oral anticoagulant with a molecular weight of 459.5 Da and is highly selective for FXa. It has a half-life of 8-15 hours and is metabolised in the liver with a small proportion excreted unchanged in the urine. Certain cautions accompany this drug, for example, patients with renal impairment should not take this drug, nor should patients taking azole antimycotics or human immunodeficiency virus protease inhibitors be prescribed apixaban [30].

Endoxaban is another selective oral inhibitor of FXa with a half-life of 7-10 hours. Absorption of endoxaban is not affected by food and is readily absorbed after oral administration [30]. Endoxaban has been used in clinical trials for the prevention of VTE and VTE in major orthopaedic surgery. Studies have shown a dose dependent reduction in the incidence of VTE when treated with endoxaban [33].

Betrixaban is a FXa inhibitor that has a half-life of 20 hours and is primarily cleared through the biliary system with minimal renal excretion [34]. It has been tested in phase II clinical trials with patients undergoing total knee replacement surgery and has shown better safety profiles when compared with enoxaparin [35]. It is also being tested and compared with enoxaparin in terms of efficacy in the treatment of patients with VTE during and post-hospitalisation [34].

Another FXa inhibitor that has been developed is darexaban, which has a rapid onset of action once it is converted to its active metabolite darexaban glucuronide upon absorption, after which it has a plasma half-life of 14-18 hours [36]. In terms of safety profiles and efficacy, darexaban compares well with enoxaparin when used as an anticoagulant in knee replacement surgery [37].

Table 3. Characteristics of a selection of Factor Xa inhibitors

FXa inhibitor	Molecular weight (Da)	Bioavailability (%)	Half-life	Primary route of clearance	Route of administration
Fondaparinux	1728	100	17-21 hours	Renal	Parenteral
Rivaroxaban	435	60-86	5-9 hours	Renal	Oral
Apixaban	459	34-88	8-15 hours	Renal	Oral
Edoxaban	548	62	7-10 hours	Renal	Oral
Darexaban	590	Unavailable	14-18 hours	Renal	Oral
Betrixaban	451	34	20 hours	Liver	Oral

Darexaban was also been evaluated in patients with atrial fibrillation and the incidence of bleeding with this drug was shown to be comparable with warfarin [35].

The major concern with FXa inhibitors is the availability of antidotes. Portola Pharmaceuticals is in the process of developing a FXa inhibitor antidote which would bind to the inhibitor and neutralise it. The efficacy of this FXa inhibitor reversal agent has been proven in preclinical studies with a mouse model, and also in animal models where it reversed the effects of enoxaparin and fondaparinux [38]. The general characteristics of selected FXa inhibitors can be seen in Table 3.

Anti-Platelet Drugs

While this chapter aims to focus on anticoagulant drugs that target FXa and thrombin, it is important to mention anti-platelet therapy in the treatment of cardiovascular disease. Platelets perform an important role in prevention of bleeding, in that they stick together to form a temporary platelet plug at the site of injury. While their actions are beneficial in some circumstances, if a blood clot develops in the brain or in the arteries or veins of the heart as a result of enhanced platelet activity, it needs to be brought under control [39]. Anti-platelet drugs interfere with platelet function and can be used in the prevention of cardiovascular disease, or used to treat acute or chronic diseases.

Aspirin, or acetylsalicylic acid, is the most widely used drug in the world, but more specifically it is the most widely used anti-platelet drug, since it was discovered in the 1960s to protect individuals from heart attacks, thus making it the gold standard antiplatelet agent [40]. Despite is important historical and widespread use, the best dose of aspirin is unknown with medics recommending approximately between 160 and 325 mg per day [39]. Aspirin is an irreversible cyclooxygenase inhibitor that prevents the production of thromboxane A_2 (TXA_2) (Figure 2) in platelets, which causes the permanent inhibition of TXA_2 for the lifespan of the platelet [4]. TXA_2 is responsible for the activation of phospholipase C and platelet aggregation, so aspirin ultimately prevents platelet aggregation [41]. Another important feature of aspirin is the fact that some people do not respond to it at all which has become known as aspirin resistance.

Clopidogrel is often administered in conjunction with aspirin to patients with angina or have had heart attacks [42]. Clopidogrel interferes with platelet stickiness, but it is a prodrug that needs to be metabolised by hepatic conversion, resulting in significant variability between patients [43]. A P2Y receptor antagonist, clopidogrel inhibits and irreversibly binds to the $P2Y_{12}$ receptor through a disulphide bridge which is important in platelet activation and fibrin cross-linking.

The inability to fully rely on aspirin and the variability of the clopidogrel effect on patients resulted in the development of new platelet antagonists. Prasugrel and ticagrelor are fast acting ADP receptor antagonists and strongly inhibit platelet activity [43]. Prasugrel irreversibly inhibits ADP-induced aggregation through the formation of a disulphide bridge between the thiol group of the active metabolite and the cysteine residue of the $P2Y_{12}$ receptor [42].

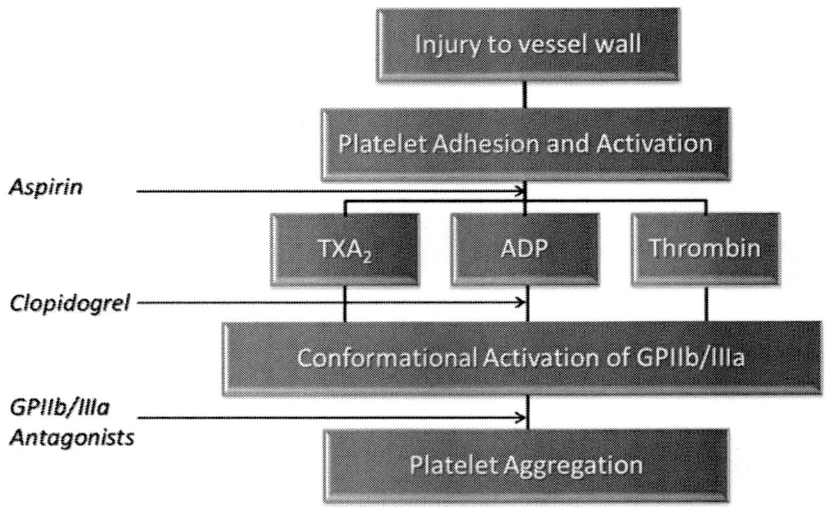

Figure 2. Targets of anti-platelet therapy. (Adapted from Jay & Lui 2006).

Ticagrelor irreversibly binds to the $P2Y_{12}$, at a site distinct from the ADP binding site, rendering it an allosteric inhibitor with a rapid onset of action and better inhibition of platelet activity than clopidogrel [44]. However, a recent publication implicated a higher incidence of bleeding after treatment with ticagrelor in cardiac surgical patients [45].

Cangrelor is a $P2Y_{12}$ inhibitor that entered clinical trials in 2009 which were halted due to disparate results, despite the rapid onset of action and the greater degree of platelet inhibition than clopidogrel. In 2013, the FDA (USA) accepted the filing for a new drug application (NDA) for cangrelor as a result of data compiled from clinical trials involving over 25,000 patients suffering from coronary artery disease [42].

Glycoprotein receptor IIb/IIIa antagonists including abciximab, aptifibatide, and tirofiban, all target these two receptors to prevent platelet aggregation [43]. Abciximab has a half-life of 12 hours and is used to reduce ischaemic complications in PCI, whereas aptifibatide, and tirofiban are about 2-4 hours. Reversing the effects of these drugs involves discontinuing the prescription.

Conclusion and Future Perspectives

While warfarin and heparin are doing the job of keeping clotting under control in affected individuals, there is a significant unmet need for a global anticoagulant that is predictable, requires little monitoring and is both safe and effective for the treatment of thromboembolic disorders. Additionally, the ideal anticoagulant will be required to be administered orally once or twice daily with immediate effect of the drug on the patient and be equally effective as heparin and warfarin in the prevention of thrombus formation [1]. In recent years there has been considerable progress in the drive and development of clinical medicine, to address the limitations of existing drugs.

Novel direct thrombin inhibitors are under development and evaluation for the prevention of VTE. One such drug being developed by AstraZeneca is AZD0837, a prodrug, that when converted to its active form, has the potential to reign superior over ximelagtran, in terms of an improved pharmacological and safety profile [23]. With a half-life of 9 hours after administration, the advantage of this drug is the fact that an extended release formulation allows for once daily administration. A comparison of AZD0837 with warfarin resulted in similar efficacy and tolerability profiles for the prevention of systemic embolism and stroke in patients with atrial fibrillation [46]. AZD0837 is currently undergoing phase III trials to determine its suitability for implementation and use as a new anticoagulant for stroke prevention.

Mousa [40] has suggested the development of recombinant protein C as an anticoagulant strategy. Protein C is a vitamin K-dependent plasma serine protease which plays a significant role in the regulation of haemostasis by hydrolytically breaking down both FVa and FVIIIa, thus preventing clot formation. The activation of protein C, in association with its cofactor protein S has the ability to inactivate activated FVa and FVIIIa. As a result this provides an anticoagulation mechanism through inhibition of thrombin generation. Recombinant protein C has been shown to improve coagulopathy in sepsis, indicating its potential usefulness as a novel strategy for anticoagulation [47].

Protein C inhibitor is a plasma glycoprotein, identified by Marlar and Griffin in 1980 [48] and while it was shown to regulate protease activated protein C, more interesting was its strong inhibitory effect on the thrombin-thrombomodulin complex [49]. With binding of thrombin to thrombomodulin, thrombin is prevented from binding to fibrinogen and from activating platelets, but thrombin will cleave protein C to form activated protein C (APC). Protein C inhibitor can therefore act as a procoagulant by inhibiting APC and an anticoagulant by inhibiting thrombin. There is thus a lot of scope here for the refinement and development of this process, whether it is chemically or genetically, to specifically target thrombin and prevent clotting.

Also highlighted by Mousa [40] is the fact that most inhibitors of coagulation have been developed to target the downstream process of the coagulation cascade such as thrombin and FXa. Blocking of factors earlier in the cascade may be more beneficial, such as tissue factor or factor VIIa.

Inhibition of FIXa has been highlighted as a potential target for the prevention of VTE. The thrombogenicity of FIXa was identified and reported as being ≈7-fold more thrombogenic than FXa and 60-fold more thrombogenic than thrombin [50]. Such reports in addition to its role in thrombin regulation have promoted FIXa as suitable target for a new anticoagulant. Two inhibitors are undergoing development including TTP889 which is a small oral molecule compound, and RB006 an injectable aptamer-based compound. Data from clinical trials with RB006 have not been published to date. However, it has been reported that TTP889 was not effective at preventing VTE in a phase II clinical trial and an additional phase II clinical trial was abandoned in 2012 [51]. Dual FXa and thrombin inhibitors that target both FXa and thrombin have been reported in the patent literature [28].

Sanofi-Aventis have disclosed 243 dual inhibitors that are equally or more potent in their inhibition of FXa compared to thrombin. A Japanese company has claimed development of amidine derivatives that act as dual FXa and thrombin inhibitors [52] and the University of North Carolina filed a patent containing data that claims the suitability of sulphated polysaccharides without iduronic acid residues, as potential FXa and thrombin antagonists [53].

While there is a continued and determined drive for the development of a pharmacologically safe, efficient and low-cost anticoagulant to prevent and treat disorders of haemostasis and coagulation, it may take many years to formulate. In addition, it will be very difficult to develop one drug that is suitable for the prevention of all indications. While the majority of the newer anticoagulants on the market have shown improvements over the traditional vitamin K antagonists or heparins, there is a clear need for robust data proving overall superiority and safety with long-term treatment. Without antidotes and simple assays to monitor new drugs, it becomes difficult to treat haemorrhagic complications. While newer drugs are being sold as not requiring coagulation monitoring, it is now believed that it would be clinically relevant to develop a simple, inexpensive and standardised test to accompany newer drugs [54]. Reduced bleeding events, fewer interactions with other medications and foods, and the reduced need for regular laboratory monitoring are all key factors that will affect the willingness of clinicians to replace standard antithrombotics with novel inhibitors in the future.

References

[1] Tsiara S, Pappas K, Boutsis D, Laffan M. New oral anticoagulants: should they replace heparins and warfarin? *Hell. J Cardiol* 2011 52, 52–67.

[2] Naess IA, Christiansen SC, Romundstad P, Cannegieter SC, Rosendaal FR, Hammerstrøm J. Incidence and mortality of venous thrombosis: a population-based study. *J. Thromb. Haemost.* 2007 5, 692–9.

[3] Cosmi B, Palareti G. Old and new heparins. *Thromb. Res.* 2012 129, 388–91.

[4] Jay RM, Lui P. How anticoagulants work. *Tech. Reg. Anesth. Pain Manag.* 2006 10, 30–9.

[5] Lassen MR, Laux V. Emergence of new oral antithrombotics: a critical appraisal of their clinical potential. *Vasc. Health Risk Manag.* 2008 4, 1373–86.

[6] Wardrop D, Keeling D. The story of the discovery of heparin and warfarin. *Br. J. Haematol.* 2008 141, 757–63.

[7] Walenga JM, Lyman GH. Evolution of heparin anticoagulants to ultra-low-molecular-weight heparins: a review of pharmacologic and clinical differences and applications in patients with cancer. *Crit. Rev. Oncol. Hematol.* 2013 88, 1–18.

[8] Hirsh J, Raschke R. Heparin and low-molecular-weight heparin - The Seventh ACCP Conference on Antithrombotic and Thrombolytic Therapy. *Chest* 2004 126, 188S–203S.

[9] Rosenberg RD. Redesigning heparin. *N. Engl. J. Med.* 2001 344, 673–5.

[10] Kelton JG, Levine MN. Heparin-Induce Thrombocytopenia. *Semin. Thromb. Haemost.* 1986 12, 59–62.

[11] Ahmed I, Majeed A, Powell R. Heparin induced thrombocytopenia: diagnosis and management update. *Postgrad. Med. J.* 2007 83, 575–82.

[12] Spyropoulos AC. Brave new world: the current and future use of novel anticoagulants. *Thromb. Res.* 2008 123, S29–35.

[13] Ignjatovic V, Najid S, Newall F, Summerhayes R, Monagle P. Dosing and monitoring of enoxaparin (Low molecular weight heparin) therapy in children. *Br. J. Haematol.* 2010 149, 734–8.

[14] Ignjatovic V, Summerhayes R, Gan A, Than J, Chan A, Cochrane A, et al. Monitoring Unfractionated Heparin (UFH) therapy: Which Anti Factor Xa assay is appropriate? *Thromb. Res.* 2007 120, 347–51.

[15] Bates SM, Weitz JI. New Antithrombotic Drugs. In: Colman RW, Marder VJ, Clowes AW, George JN, Goldhaber S, editor. Hemostasis and Thrombosis: Basic Principles and Clinical Practice, Philadelphia, USA: Lippincott Williams & Wilkins; 2006, p. 1763.

[16] Greinacher A, Warkentin TE. The direct thrombin inhibitor hirudin. *Thromb. Haemost.* 2008 99, 819–29.

[17] Hirsh J, O'Donnell M, Weitz JI. New anticoagulants. *Blood* 2005 105, 453–63.

[18] Hogg PJ, Jackson CM. Fibrin monomer protects thrombin from inactivation by heparin-AT 3. Implications for heparin efficiency,. *Proc. Natl. Acad. Sci. U. S. A.* 1989 86, 3619–23.

[19] Weitz JI, Hudoba M, D Ma, Maraganore J, Hirsh J. Clot-bound thrombin is protected from inhibition by heparin-AT III but is susceptible to

inactivation by antithroimbin-III-independent inhibitors. *J. Clincal Investig.* 1990 86, 385–91.
[20] Chong BH. Heparin-induced thrombocytopenia. *J. Thromb. Haemost.* 2003 1, 1471–8.
[21] Ten Y, Devlin G. Bivalirudin in acute coronary syndromes and percutaneous coronary intervention: should we use it? *Heart Lung Circ.* 2013 22, 793–800.
[22] Weitz JI, Bates SM. Beyond Heparin and Aspirin. *Arch. Intern. Med.* 2000 160, 749.
[23] Lee CJ, Ansell JE. Direct thrombin inhibitors. *Br. J. Clin. Pharmacol.* 2011 72, 581–92.
[24] Desai J, Granger CB, Weitz JI, Aisenberg J. Novel oral anticoagulants in gastroenterology practice. *Gastrointest. Endosc.* 2013 78, 227–39.
[25] Stangier J, Rathgen K, Stähle H, Gansser D, Roth W. The pharmacokinetics, pharmacodynamics and tolerability of dabigatran etexilate, a new oral direct thrombin inhibitor, in healthy male subjects. *Br. J. Clin. Pharmacol.* 2007 64, 292–303.
[26] Bates SM, Weitz JI. Coagulation assays. *Circulation* 2005 112, e53–60.
[27] Wittkowsky A. New oral anticoagulants. In: Dager W, Gulseth M, Nutescu E, editors. Anticoagulation Therapy: A Point-of-Care Guide, Maryland, USA: American Society of Health-System Pharmacists; 2011, p. 181.
[28] Pinto DJP, Qiao JX, Knabb RM. The emergence of factor Xa inhibitors for the treatment of cardiovascular diseases: a patent review. *Expert Opin. Ther. Pat.* 2012; 22, 645–61.
[29] Di Nisio M, Buller H. Antithrombotic therapy in venous thrombosis and pulmonary embolism. In: Moliterno DJ, Kristensen Steen D, De Caterina Raffaele, editors. Therapeutic Advances in Thrombosis, Sussex, UK.: John Wiley & Sons; 2012, p. 400.
[30] De Caterina R, Husted S, Wallentin L, Andreotti F, Arnesen H, Bachmann F, et al. New oral anticoagulants in atrial fibrillation and acute coronary syndromes: ESC Working Group on Thrombosis-Task Force on Anticoagulants in Heart Disease position paper. *J. Am. Coll. Cardiol.* 2012 59, 1413–25.
[31] Kakkar AK, Brenner B, Dahl OE, Eriksson BI, Mouret P, Muntz J, et al. Extended duration rivaroxaban versus short-term enoxaparin for the prevention of venous thromboembolism after total hip arthroplasty: a double-blind, randomised controlled trial. *Lancet* 2008 372, 31–9.

[32] Thomas TF, Ganetsky V, Spinler SA. Rivaroxaban: an oral factor Xa inhibitor. *Clin. Ther.* 2013 35, 4–27.

[33] Becattini C, Vedovati MC, Agnelli G. Old and new oral anticoagulants for venous thromboembolism and atrial fibrillation: a review of the literature. *Thromb. Res.* 2012 129, 392–400.

[34] Ahrens I, Peter K, Lip GYH, Bode C. Development and Clinical Applications of Novel Oral Anticoagulants. Part II. Drugs Under Clinical Investigation. *Discov. Med.* 2012 13, 445–50.

[35] Turpie AGG, Bauer KA, Davidson BL, Fisher WD, Gent M, Huo MH, et al. A randomized evaluation of betrixaban, an oral factor Xa inhibitor, for prevention of thromboembolic events after total knee replacement (EXPERT). *Thromb. Haemost.* 2009 101, 68–76.

[36] Iwatsuki Y, Sato T, Moritani Y, Shigenaga T, Suzuki M, Kawasaki T, et al. Biochemical and pharmacological profile of darexaban, an oral direct factor Xa inhibitor. *Eur. J. Pharmacol.* 2011 673, 49–55.

[37] Ahrens I, Lip GY, Peter K. New oral anticoagulant drugs in cardiovascular disease. *Thromb. Haemost.* 2010 104, 49–60.

[38] Lu G, Deguzman F, Karbarz M, Hollenbach S, Conley P, Hutchaleelaha A, et al. Reversal of rivaroxaban mediated anticoagulation in animal models by a recombinant antidote protein (r-Antidote, PRT064445). *Eur. Hear J.* 2011 32, 640–1.

[39] Harrington RA, Hodgson PK, Larsen RL. Cardiology patient page. Antiplatelet therapy. *Circulation* 2003 108, e45–7.

[40] Mousa S. Highlights of latest advances in antithrombotics. In: Mousa S, editor. Anticoagulants, Antiplatelets, and Thrombolytics, New Jersey, USA: Humana Press Inc.; 2004, p. 6.

[41] Floyd CN, Ferro A. Mechanisms of aspirin resistance. *Pharmacol. Ther.* 2014 141, 69–78.

[42] Yeung J, Holinstat M. Newer agents in antiplatelet therapy: a review. *J. Blood Med.* 2012 3, 33–42.

[43] Yorkgitis BK, Ruggia-Check C, Dujon JE. Antiplatelet and anticoagulation medications and the surgical patient. *Am. J. Surg.* 2014 207, 95–101.

[44] Wallentin L, Becker RC, Budaj A, Cannon CP, Emanuelsson H, Held C, et al. Ticagrelor versus clopidogrel in patients with acute coronary syndromes. *N. Engl. J. Med.* 2009 361, 1045–57.

[45] Schotola H, Bräuer A, Meyer K, Hinz J, Schöndube FA, Bauer M, et al. Perioperative outcomes of cardiac surgery patients with ongoing

ticagrelor therapy: boon and bane of a new drug. *Eur. J. Cardiothorac. Surg.* 2014 doi: 10.1093/ejcts/ezt571.

[46] Olsson SB, Rasmussen LH, Tveit A, Jensen E, Wessman P, Panfilov S, et al. Safety and tolerability of an immediate-release formulation of theoral direct thrombin inhibitor AZD0837 in the prevention of stroke and systemic embolism in patients with atrial fibrillation. *Thromb. Haemost.* 2010 103, 604–12.

[47] Kazmi RS, Lwaleed BA. New anticoagulants: how to deal with treatment failure and bleeding complications. *Br. J. Clin. Pharmacol.* 2011 72, 593–603.

[48] Marlar R a, Griffin JH. Deficiency of protein C inhibitor in combined factor V/VIII deficiency disease. *J. Clin. Invest.* 1980 66, 1186–9.

[49] Elisen MG, von dem Borne P a, Bouma BN, Meijers JC. Protein C inhibitor acts as a procoagulant by inhibiting the thrombomodulin-induced activation of protein C in human plasma. *Blood* 1998 91, 1542–7.

[50] Gitel SN, Stephenson RC, Wessler S. In vitro and in vivo correlation of clotting protease activity: effect of heparin. *Proc. Natl. Acad. Sci. U. S. A.* 1977 74, 3028–32.

[51] Eriksson BI, Dahl OE, Lassen MR, Ward DP, Rothlein R, Davis G, et al. Partial factor IXa inhibition with TTP889 for prevention of venous thromboembolism: an exploratory study. *J. Thromb. Haemost.* 2008 6, 457–63.

[52] Fukuda Y, Kayahara T, Nakagawa T, Sagi K, Shoji M, Takahara A, et al. Benzamidine derivative. WO1999064392 A1, 1999.

[53] Liu J, Hill C, Nc US, Jones C. Enzymatic synthesis of sulfated polysaccharides without iduronic acid residues. US 2009/0035787 A1, 2009.

[54] Weitz JI, Hirsh J, Samama MM. New anticoagulant drugs: the 8th ACCP Conference on Antithrombotic and Thrombolytic Therapy. *Chest* 2008 133,234S-256S.

In: Heparin
Editor: Nicole B. Wilkinson
ISBN: 978-1-63117-624-1

Chapter III

Heparin and Vascular Health

Linda Hiebert[1,*] and Jimin Liu[2]
[1]Department of Veterinary Biomedical Sciences,
University of Saskatchewan, Saskatoon, Canada
[2]Department of Pathology and Molecular Medicine,
McMaster University, Hamilton, Canada

Abstract

Heparin is a highly negatively charged heterogeneous compound, derived from animal tissue that has been used as an antithrombotic drug for more than 70 years. It is generally believed that the efficacy of heparin as an antithrombotic agent is primarily due to its anticoagulant mechanism where it acts to catalyze antithrombin III and heparin cofactor II, natural inhibitors of activated coagulation factors. However, because of its negative charge, administered heparins bind to many cationic molecules present in the circulation and on the vessel wall, particularly the endothelium. There is considerable evidence that the interaction of heparins with the vessel wall not only contributes to the antithrombotic effects of heparins but may be important in preventing vascular disorders thus contributing to vascular health. There is evidence that the interaction of heparin and heparin-like compounds with the vasculature, may be of

* Corresponding Author: Linda Hiebert Ph.D., Department of Veterinary Biomedical Sciences, University of Saskatchewan, Saskatoon, Saskatchewan, S7N 5B4 Canada. Phone: 306 966 7358, Fax 306 966 7376. Email:linda.hiebert@usask.ca.

benefit in the prevention and treatment of atherosclerosis and its complications. The continued successful application of heparin in the design and engineering of stents used for the treatment of atherosclerosis underlines the important role that this drug plays in the health of the vessel wall. Thus the interaction of heparin and related compounds with the blood vessels may contribute to vascular health and have benefits that require further exploration and development.

Heparins and Heparan Sulfates

Heparin is a naturally occurring compound belonging to the glycosaminoglycan (GAG) family. In addition to heparin the GAGs include heparan sulfate, chondroitin sulfate, dermatan sulfate, keratan sulfate and hyaluronan. The GAGs are part of large heterogeneous molecules known as the proteoglycans which consist of a protein core with one or more GAG covalently attached. Proteoglycans are produced by all cells and can be found in secretory granules, cell membranes or in the surrounding extracellular environment as a result of cell secretion or shedding from the cell membrane [1]. Chemically, GAGs are linear carbohydrate chains consisting of repeating units of disaccharides composed of a uronic acid moiety (D-glucuronic or L-iduronic acid) and an amino sugar (D-galactosamine or D-glucosamine), except for keratan sulfate which contains repeating units of glucosamine and galactosamine. The amino sugars can be N-acetylated and sulfated and the uronic acid moiety sulfated, which impart a high negative charge to the molecules and ensure linearity. GAGs are diverse in chain length, disaccharide content, and disaccharide modifications such as degree of sulfation resulting in variation in charge density.

Heparin is the GAG that has the highest charge density. Heparin is produced by the mast cell as part of the serglycin molecule. Serglycin is a small proteoglycan, found in mast cell granules, whose GAG component is highly negatively charged such as heparin or chondroitin sulfate [2]. The GAGs attached to serglycin help bind granules of a basic nature such as biogenic amines, including histamine and serotonin, cytokines, and proteases such as chymase, tryptase and carboxypeptidases. Thus it is believed that serglycin with attached heparin GAGs help stabilize the mast cell granule and its contents.

Heparin has traditionally been prepared from animal tissue particularly from porcine or bovine mucosal or lung tissue. As a prepared drug, unfractionated heparin (UFH) is a negatively charged polyanion with a core disaccharide structure of →4)-α-D-glucosamine-2,6-disulfate (1→4)-α-iduronic acid-2-sulfate (1→. The disaccharide units are variable; glucuronic acid may replace iduronic acid, N–acetyl may replace N–sulfate groups, and O-sulfate groups may be absent. Variation also exists in the degree of polymerization so that in a single preparation of UFH, chain lengths vary from 10 to 80 disaccharide units [3] with molecular weights ranging from 2-40 kD, and mean molecular weights varying from 12-16 kD [4]. Derivatives of UFH, the low molecular weight heparins (LMWHs), have been developed using nitrous acid degradation, benzylation-alkaline hydrolysis, peroxidative cleavage or heparinase, etc. LMWHs have a mean molecular weight of 4-7 kD [4]. Although each LMWH is chemically unique they have less protein binding, increased bioavailability, a more predictable dose response and a longer pharmacodynamic half-life than UFH on subcutaneous administration [5,6]. Recently a synthetic pentasaccharide, a structure characterizing a molecular sequence in heparin that has anticoagulant activity, has gained approval for clinical use as an anticoagulant. Techniques to simplify production of this specific pentasaccharide and reduce production costs, using a chemoenzymatic process, are currently under investigation [7].

Heparin is similar in structure and function to heparan sulfate, a GAG found as part of heparan sulfate proteoglycans (HSPGs) in the extracellular matrix and on many cells including endothelial cells [8]. Chemically, heparan sulfate consists of repeating units of glucuronic acid and acetylated glucosamine where diversity in structure is largely due to the replacement of uronic acid by iduronic acid and by variability in the degree of sulfation. Heparan sulfate molecules can consist of 48 different disaccharide building blocks [9]. A structure activity relationship likely exists for the various heparan sulfate structures [10]. Like heparin, heparan sulfate is highly negatively charged, binds to and may alter activity of many cationic molecules [11]. Syndecan and glypican are HSPGs associated with the endothelial plasma membrane while the HSPG perlecan is found in the basement membrane of most endothelial cells [12]. Important regulatory proteins that bind to heparan sulfate include bFGF, lipoprotein lipase (LPL), hepatic lipase, antithrombin III, Apo B and Apo E, superoxide dismutase (SOD) and selectins [13]. Heparan sulfate is the shear stress receptor for nitric oxide release which results in relaxation of the underlying smooth muscles of blood vessels resulting in vasodilation [14]. As well, heparan sulfate plays a role in fat metabolism where in the liver, chylomicron remnants bind to HSPGs allowing transfer to receptors followed by uptake by the hepatocytes [15].

Because of their polyanionic nature, heparin and heparan sulfates interact with a wide variety of proteins, the most studied being those responsible for anticoagulant activity. A specific pentasaccharide sequence in heparin and heparan sulfate activate antithrombin III, which inhibits many activated coagulation factors, most importantly factor Xa; and heparin cofactor II, an inhibitor of thrombin but also factor Xa. About one-third of UFH chains have the specific pentasaccharide sequence with high affinity for antithrombin III, with only one or two pentasaccharide groups per chain making up about 5% of the total UFH preparation [16, 17]. Heparin chains of less than 24 monosaccharide units are not able to bind to heparin cofactor II, thus their anticoagulant effect is only through antithrombin III activation. LMWHs therefore have a higher anti-factor Xa/IIa ratio than UFH. The activated partial thromboplastin time (APTT), used to monitor UFH, is not very effective in measuring LMWH and therefore anti-factor Xa activity is used [18]. However, correlation between APTT or anti-Xa activity and antithrombotic activity remains questionable [19, 20]. Release of tissue factor pathway inhibitor (TFPI) from endothelium by heparin may also contribute to heparin's anticoagulant activity *in vivo* [21, 22].

The Blood Vessels

The blood vessels can be divided into the arteries, capillaries and veins. The arteries are a common location of vascular disease and are the sites of arteriosclerosis, aortic aneurysms, stroke, peripheral arterial disease, etc. The basic functions of arteries are to supply blood to the organs and maintain blood pressure. Depending on the size and location, arteries can be divided into three types: large (or elastic arteries), i.e. aorta; medium-sized (or muscular arteries), i.e. coronary arteries; and small arteries/arterioles, i.e. those located within the organs. The arteries are composed of three layers: intima, media and adventitia, which are more delineated in the large arteries. The intima includes the monolayer of endothelial cells and subendothelial connective tissue. The media is mainly composed of smooth muscle cells with a large amount of extracellular matrix and some elastic tissue, in particular the internal elastic lamina and external elastic lamina in the large/elastic arteries. The adventitia is the outer covering of the blood vessels and is composed of loose connective tissue but also fibroblasts, mast cells, macrophages, ganglionic cells, immunomodulatory cells, resident progenitor cells, vasa vasorum endothelial cells, and adrenergic nerves. It functions to support the blood vessel but also is a scaffold for sympathetic nerve endings and small arterioles, named the vasa vasorum. The blood supply of the large elastic arteries is from two different sources; the intima and the inner smooth muscle cells are nourished by direct diffusion from the lumen, while the outer smooth muscle cells and adventitia are supplied by the vasa vasorum. The veins are thinner and more collapsible than the arteries. They contain an intima as in arteries but the media is poorly developed with some smooth muscle and elastic fibres while the adventitia is made of loose connective tissue and vascular myoblast–type cells. The veins have valves that allow only one way flow. The veins collect blood from the capillaries and offer some exchange between blood and tissues, return blood to the heart but also are a prime storage site of blood in the circulation. The veins are the most common site of thrombosis.

Endothelium

The endothelium is a distributed organ consisting of a monolayer of cells found on the lumenal surface of all blood vessels and lymphatics. The endothelial cells are variable in structure and function [23]. Variation depends on the organ, type of vessel, and its interaction with the extracellular environment so that the endothelium adapts itself to the environment of each organ and to different conditions within the organ. There are also species differences between endothelium. The age of endothelial cells also affect their functions, for example, aging of endothelial cells is associated with decreased nitric oxide synthesis and increased sensitivity to apoptosis [24].

The endothelium performs many functions that sustain the health of the organism. The endothelium regulates fluid exchange between the blood and interstitial fluid (reviewed in [25]). It regulates vascular tone of the blood vessels by affecting the underlying smooth muscle with the appropriate release of nitric oxide, prostacyclin, endothelium derived hyperpolarizing factor and endothelin. It synthesizes many important components including coagulation factors, tissue plasminogen activator, connective tissue components such as collagen and elastin, and proteoglycans. Many compounds within the circulating blood such as adenosine, bradykinin, angiotensin I and II, serotonin, endorphins, substance P, histamine, etc., are metabolized by endothelium. It participates in inflammatory responses where it influences leukocyte trafficking particularly in post capillary venules. It maintains a non-thrombogenic surface but can also promote thrombosis when injured. The endothelium separates the blood from underlying components of the vessel wall which, if exposed, can result in leukocyte and platelet activation and stimulation of the coagulation mechanism. The endothelium not only serves as a target for cytokines but can express many pro and anti-inflammatory cytokines when activated [26]

A meshwork of proteoglycans and glycoproteins known as the glycocalyx covers the surface of endothelial cells with most components attached to the plasma membrane [27]. The glycocalyx is negatively charged largely due to the presence of GAGs including heparan sulfate, chondroitin sulfate and hyaluronan which is secreted by endothelial cells and becomes bound by receptors on the endothelial cell membrane [28]. Heparan sulfate, as part of the proteoglycans on the endothelial surface, enhance the activity of antithrombin thus preventing coagulation. Heparan sulfate also plays a role in cell recognition, growth factor signaling and cell adhesion. Negative charges on the luminal surface of endothelial cells are also important for controlling vascular permeability by acting as a "charge barrier" to the transvascular movement of anionic plasma proteins, such as albumin [29]. In the kidney, the glomerular filter consists of fenestrated endothelium and foot processes of epithelial cells called podocytes between which is a unique glomerular basement membrane. HSPGs such as agrin and perlecan are integral parts of this glomerular basement membrane which help prevent movement of anionic charged and large molecules through the filter [30, 31].Also at this site HS may be a storage depot for growth factors such as PDGF, bFGF, hepatocyte growth factor and platelet factor 4; perform an anticoagulant function; and inhibit mesangial proliferation [32].

Vascular Smooth Muscle

Smooth muscle cells constitute the media of blood vessels, facilitate the distribution of blood among all organs, regulate vascular tone-diameter and control blood pressure. During embryonic development, the mesoderm-derived endothelial cells initially form connected channels. Later, at birth, additional supporting layers of smooth muscle cells, elastin and fibrous tissue are developed around the endothelial channels.

Based on both *in vitro* and *in vivo* morphology studies, smooth muscle cells can be divided into two phenotypes, synthetic and contractile [33]. The synthetic phenotype is often seen in embryonic development, and in injury-related or diseased conditions. These smooth muscle cells are capable of proliferation and migration, and often produce large amounts of extracellular matrix. The contractile type of smooth muscle cell is present and functional in adult or mature vessels. These smooth muscle cells express more contractile proteins than the synthetic phenotype which include smooth muscle myosin heavy chain, smooth muscle α-actin, h-caldesmon and calponin. The contractile muscle cells also express surface receptors, ion channels or regulating proteins and signal transduction molecules. These smooth muscle cells are less proliferative and produce a smaller amount of extracellular matrix than the synthetic cells.

One of the unique features of vascular smooth muscle cells is the ability to switch phenotype depending on the local microenvironment. For example, in normal adults, vascular smooth muscle cells display the contractile phenotype. During injury, for example in endothelial damage or post percutaneous transluminal coronary angioplasty (PTCA), vascular smooth muscle cells express the synthetic phenotype that are able to migrate, proliferate and produce large amount of extracellular matrix. When the endothelium returns to intact status, the underlying smooth muscle cells will regain their contractile phenotype and continue their normal vascular functions, i.e. regulation of blood pressure. In summary, vascular smooth muscle cells play a critical role in normal vascular physiology.

There are several pathological conditions related to vascular smooth muscle cells, i.e. atherosclerosis, restenosis in post-PTCA therapy, arteriosclerosis in graft rejection, and hypertension. In atherosclerosis, the affected arteries show a thickened wall with a collection of smooth muscle cells, foamy histiocytes, inflammatory cells and a lipid core. The key features in the pathogenesis of atherosclerosis are endothelial injury and smooth muscle cell proliferation. The intact layer of endothelium has a protective effect on smooth muscles and prevents smooth muscle cell proliferation.

Heparin Interaction with Endothelium

Because of its high charge, heparin interacts with the vascular wall, formed elements and plasma proteins [34]. UFHs are avidly taken up by endothelial cells when added to medium [35-42], applied to the aortic lumenal surface [43] or when given *in vivo* [44-47]. In initial studies we observed an increase in ruthenium red staining on the surface of endothelial cells by electron microscopy, suggesting an increase in the thickness of the glycocalyx, five minutes following intravenous administration of 1000 units of heparin to rats compared to rats injected with saline [44]. Internalization by endothelium with possible incorporation into lysosomes, evidence of degradation and release into cell medium has been observed [42, 48, 49]. LMWHs are also bound and internalized by endothelium [6, 38, 50] although with less affinity than UFH. Heparin binds to endothelial cell growth factors and modulates angiogenesis mediated by other agents [51-53]. Heparin releases lipoprotein lipase (LPL) [54], diamine oxidase [55], extracellular superoxide dismutase [56], platelet factor 4 [57], and TFPI [21] from the endothelial surface into the circulation.

There is considerable evidence that heparins are protective of endothelium. Our work has also revealed that GAGs and related polyanions prevent endothelial cell injury from reactive oxygen species (ROS) [58-60] and high glucose [61, 62]. Polycationic substances, including protamine, increased vascular permeability in isolated rat lungs, but the presence of heparin reduced this effect [63].

Evidence exists that heparin administration increases heparan sulfate synthesis in both rabbit and human endothelial cells [64, 65]. Heparin suppresses production of endothelin, a vasoconstrictor [66]. Heparin has many anti-inflammatory activities (reviewed in [67]). Heparins interfere with recruitment of leukocytes by the vascular wall, block the adhesion molecules L- and P-selectins [68], bind to Mac-1 thus inhibiting neutrophil adhesion to endothelial cells [69] and inhibit release of elastase from neutrophils [70]. Heparin inhibits NF-κB translocation from cytoplasm to nucleus of human endothelial cells [71] and T cells [72]. Thus, in addition to antithrombotic and anticoagulant effects, heparins have many additional benefits that are largely unexplored.

Heparin and Smooth Muscle

Considerable evidence has shown that heparin inhibits smooth muscle cell proliferation [73-76]. In 1977, Clowes and Karnovsky using a rat carotid artery endothelial injury model demonstrated that exogenous heparin inhibited smooth muscle cell proliferation [73]. Proliferation of cultured smooth muscle cells derived from Sprague-Dawley rat aorta were inhibited by heparin with both anticoagulant and non-anticoagulant heparins being effective [77]. To further prove the inhibitory function shown in the above findings, heparin-like material was identified in the conditioned medium from confluent cultured endothelium [78]. In a different experiment, using bovine aortic smooth muscle cultures, Fritze identified an inhibitory factor (heparan sulfate) secreted by confluent smooth muscle cells [79]. This factor was able to reduce the growth rate of the cultured smooth muscle cells. Heparin and related GAGs similarly prevented the proliferation of fetal bovine serum stimulated division of bovine trachealis smooth muscle cells [80]. A heparan sulfate proteoglycan, derived from basement membrane of endothelial cells cultured from fetal bovine pulmonary arteries, inhibited smooth muscle proliferation [81]. Therefore heparin and heparan sulfate, either exogenous or endogenous, is able to reduce smooth muscle cell proliferation and decrease the consequences of vascular injury.

Heparin and Thrombosis

Heparin has been used as an antithrombotic drug since its initial use in 1935 [82]. The antithrombotic action of heparin is largely attributed to its anticoagulant activity where it activates antithrombin III and heparin cofactor II. However there is much evidence that the interaction of heparin with endothelium may be largely responsible for the antithrombotic activity of heparin. Binding to endothelium markedly increases antithrombotic activity such that heparin need not be in blood to be an effective antithrombotic agent [83].

To prevent thrombosis, heparins are given primarily by intravenous and subcutaneous routes. It is generally assumed that heparins are not effective when given orally based on the beliefs that 1) the high negative charge and size of the heparin molecule make it unsuitable for absorption, 2) low pH and digestive enzymes of the stomach may degrade heparin [84], and 3) little or no change in anticoagulant activity is observed following oral heparin administration [85]. However, our own studies concerning the antithrombotic effects of orally administered heparin in a rat jugular vein model have shown that thrombosis was prevented by oral UFHs [86], and LMWHs when the vessel was examined 4 h after initiation of thrombosis and drug administration [87]. A dose-dependent decrease in thrombosis was observed with oral UFH [86, 87], and the LMWHs tinzaparin and reviparin [87-89]. Orally administered LMWHs were effective at lower doses than UFH suggesting that LMWHs may be absorbed faster than UFH. In the rat jugular vein thrombosis model ED_{50}s of 7.5, 0.1 and 0.025 mg/kg were seen for UFH, tinzaparin and reviparin, respectively [87-89]. Similarly we have shown that thrombosis was prevented by oral heparins in a rat carotid artery model [90] and in a rat venous stasis model [91]. In these studies, we demonstrated that heparin could be found associated with endothelium even though there were minimal amounts of chemical heparin found in plasma and little or no evidence of anticoagulant activity [46, 47, 87, 92]. Additionally in our studies, subcutaneous heparin, used as a control for oral administration, showed similar antithrombotic activity as oral heparin administration despite little or no change in anticoagulant activity [93]; largely suggesting that binding to endothelium is as important as anticoagulant activity in preventing thrombosis.

In a human study, ninety-seven subjects with unstable angina, were given orally, on a daily basis, 10,000 units of porcine intestinal mucosal heparin in combination with arginine (3.3 gms orally) for 12 months. The cardiac event rates, observed at 12 months post diagnosis of angina, showed a dramatic significant reduction in myocardial infarction, readmission and revascularization when compared to those of a FRISC II trial (23) [94]. There was no evidence of gastrointestinal irritation in these subjects. These studies indicate that oral administration of heparin may be suitable in long term studies in the clinical setting to sustain vascular health.

Heparin and Atherosclerosis

Many previous studies have suggested and observed that heparin may be important in the treatment and prevention of atherosclerosis (reviewed in [95-97]). These suggestions were based on observations that serum cholesterol and lipoprotein levels were inversely correlated with endogenous plasma heparin levels, that heparin bound to and was protective of endothelium, and that heparins were observed to have anti-inflammatory activity including the inhibition of complement, and antioxidant ability. Additionally heparin inhibits smooth muscle cell proliferation and has been observed to reduce the size of plaques in injured rat carotid arteries [73]. Previous studies have shown that heparan sulfate and NO are reduced in the atherosclerotic process [98] thus the ability of administered heparin to restore heparan sulfate levels may be of benefit [99]. As well, heparin has been reported to enhance the recovery of NO generation after injury to rabbit aorta [100]. Hunt outlines the usefulness of LMWH as an alternative to UFH in the treatment of acute coronary syndromes associated with arterial atherosclerosis, although there was little evidence to support the use of LMWH in the treatment of stroke [101]. However recently, the Fraxiparin in Stroke Study for the Treatment of Ischemic Stroke (FISS-tris) trial compared LMWH with aspirin in patients with acute ischemic stroke or large artery occlusive disease. Analysis of subgroups showed that the LMWH nadroparn calcium was superior to aspirin in patients over sixty-eight, without ongoing platelet therapy on admission, and in patients with posterior circulation stroke although there was no over-all superiority in the use of LMWH compared to aspirin in the Barthel Index score which was the primary endpoint [102].

Heparin and Restenosis

Recent advances in understanding the molecular basis of atherosclerosis and the effects of heparin on both arterial endothelial cells and smooth muscle cells bring new insights concerning the management of patients with arteriosclerosis. The overall treatment regimen for ischemic heart disease patients includes; changing life style; controlling underlying medical disorders, i.e. hyperlipidemia, diabetes, hypertension; and intervention procedures, i.e. PTCA and coronary artery bypass. In this discussion we focus on the preventive measures used in the control of arterial restenosis after angioplasty or other types of invasive procedures that affect the vessel wall.

PTCA and stent placement are the two main intravascular interventions for the management of atherosclerosis. With this procedure a catheter is inserted to dilate the artery mechanically, break down the atherosclerotic cap and restore vascular flow. When needed, a stent can be implanted at the dilated site to protect the artery. Stents are tube-like structures and most are made of expandable metal mesh. Recently, bioabsorbable stents have become available, which play the same initial role as the conventional ones and but slowly lose the stent backbone with time.

Within the arteries, the stent struts anchor to the arterial wall directly, to support the vessels. Both the PTCA procedure itself and the implanted stents will cause some pathological changes in the arteries. After the intervention, the endothelial cells are denuded, and the underlying smooth muscle cells are injured. Wound healing is initiated immediately and reendothelialization of the artery takes place. Most patients recover well after PTCA. However, due to pre-existing medical conditions and procedure induced injuries (i.e. arterial wall tear), healing may be complicated and prolonged.

Sudden vascular reclosure is the most common and life threatening complication in early post-catheterization therapy [103]. It often occurs within one month of the therapy and is related to either vascular wall damage or intraluminal thrombosis. As a part of normal healing, after the above initial phase, smooth muscle cells from the media or circulating progenitor cells migrate to the intima and undergo proliferation, which peak in the initial few months after PCTA. In about 6 month after PTCA, the proliferative intima undergoes regression, which will be eventually replaced by a layer of fibrous tissue. However, in about 30-40% of patients there is an excessive proliferation of the smooth muscle cells with an exuberant amount of ECM, which results in arterial restenosis [104]. Clinically, these patients often require a second PTCA. In addition to the proliferation of the intimal smooth muscle cells, intraluminal thrombosis also contributes to this complication [103].

PTCA was first introduced for human use in 1977 by Gruntzig [105]. The application of PTCA dramatically increased survival rate in patients with ischemic heart disease [106]. However, arterial elastic recoil (sudden luminal occlusion) and early onset of restenosis were the two main complications observed in long term follow-up. In 1987 an intravascular self-expandable stainless-steel prosthesis, or 'bare-metal stents' (BMS) were introduced [106]. This device was able to prevent elastic recoil of the injured arteries and further improve the survival rate compared with angioplasty alone [106, 107]. The side effects associated with BMS, in long term follow-up data, included in-stent restenosis and stent thrombosis. To eliminate these complications, drug-eluting stents, coated with different medications for local delivery were introduced for patients in clinical trials. The first two medications selected for study were an antiproliferative agent - paclitaxel and an immunosuppressor – sirolimus (rapamycin) [108, 109], both approved by the US Food and Drug Administration (FDA) for general use. The drug-eluting stents displayed a reduced incidence of early onset restenosis and other complications compared to that of BMS [110]. However, chronic endothelial injury, thrombosis, chronic inflammation and cytokine release at the stent site all contributed to late onset restenosis. To further explore or control these side effects, different types of drug delivery devices were developed, i.e. dual drug-eluting stents (adding an antithrombotic agent), biodegradable stents [111, 112], and drug-eluting balloons [113].

Komatsu first reported arterial changes in patients with BMS placement [114]. As early as 9 days after procedure, there were collections of fibrin, macrophages and some spindle cells around the stent struts. In 64 days after the procedure, the stents were totally encapsulated by a circumferential layer of neointima. The neointima is composed of proliferative smooth muscle cells, inflammatory cells, macrophages, and an abundance of extracellular matrix covered by a layer of endothelium. In most patients this layer of neointima regresses to a thin layer in about one year after the initial procedure. However, in some patients, this layer gets thicker and eventually results in in-stent restenosis. Depending on clinical symptoms and the degree of stenosis, patients often require an additional intervention.

Neoatherosclerosis is a terminology used to describe a form of atherosclerosis which occurs on the luminal surface of the neointima in post-stented patients several years after the initial procedure. Similar to the development of atherosclerosis in de novo arteries, the pathogenesis of neoatherosclerosis is mainly related to the endothelial damage in stented arteries [115], intravascular thrombosis, direct mechanical injury from the stent [116-119] and a local tissue inflammatory reaction to the placed stent [120], the most important being delayed reendothelialization and thrombosis.

In contrast to BMS, drug-eluting stents, with the addition of antiproliferative agents i.e. placlitaxel or sirolimus/tacrolimus, have less risk of developing restenosis secondary to reduced smooth muscle proliferation. However, delayed endothelial healing and its associated thrombosis were observed in this type of stent in a two year follow-up study [121].

Alternatively, bioabsorbable stents with eluting medication came into clinical use and have proven to have less effect on vascular restenosis and long term neoatherosclerosis [122, 123].

Heparin-Coated Metal Stents

Because of stent related intravascular thrombosis and restenosis, efforts were made to either improve the surface quality of the stent or coat the stent with different types of thromboresistant materials, i.e. hydrogels, polyurethanes, etc. After several years of animal experiments, in 1996, for the first time, a multicentric randomized study was conducted to compare the clinical outcome of the heparin coated Palmaz-Schats stent plus antiplatelet therapy with PTCA alone in elective patients with coronary artery atherosclerosis (named Benestent-II Pilot Study, [124, 125]). In 6 and 12 month follow-up, the heparin-coated stent was proven to be safe and patients with this device had no incidence of (sub) acute stent-related thrombosis and had a low incidence of restenosis. However, this trial was limited due to the comparison of two different interventions i.e. with the addition of an antiplatelet agent in one group.

The heparin-coated Wiktor stent was used in another unrandomized multicentric clinical trial from 1996 to 1997, which involved 132 patients [126]. All patients were given heparin-coated Wiktor stents and observed for 12 month for the incidence of thrombosis and restenosis. The final results revealed that the incidence of subacute thrombosis was low. However, the incidence of restenosis remained the same.

In 2001, patients with a different type of stent (Jostent) were enrolled in a randomized clinical trial [127]. All 277 patients were divided into two groups for either heparin-coated or uncoated stents. In 6 month follow-up, the results did not reveal any significant difference between the two groups in terms of stent related thrombosis and restenosis.

In numerous animal studies, heparin has been proven to be an antithrombotic agent, a smooth muscle cell proliferative inhibitor and an endothelial recovering modulator. However, the results from the clinical trials above seemed to be controversial and inclusive. Could a bioabsorbable stent (a transient /temporary stent) or a bioabsorbable stent loaded with heparin or other medications be able to solve the above dilemma and restore vascular function?

Bioabsorbable Stents and Vascular Restoration (Tissue Engineering)

At the time when metal stents were used in clinical trials and services, the bioabsorbable stent was still in its infancy. Because of the obstacle in selecting suitable biocompatible materials, there was an initial delay in the development of this type of stent. An ideal bioabsorbable stent should be made of a fully bioabsorbable scaffold, which was able to provide the vascular support in the initial post-PTCA phase, elute a built-in medication when needed and disappear from the site when the healing was completed. Compared with the metal stent, the bioabsorbable stent should have less adverse effects on the implanted vessels, deliver sustained medications or genes locally and restore the vascular structure to full function.

In 1998, for the first time, a type of biodegradable poly-l-lactic acid (PLLA) stents (named PLLA Igaki-Tamai stent) were implanted in the coronary arteries of a small group of selected patients [128]. Both early and at 6 month follow-up, the stent was proven to be safe and there was no stent related early thrombosis nor vascular recoil and restenosis. Subsequently, more patients were enrolled in the study using the same type of PLLA stent [129]. The 10 year follow-up results proved Igaki-Tamai stents were safe, had similar clinical protective effects in post-PTCA patients as in bare-metal stented patients and showed less long term stent related thrombosis and restenosis. Based on intravascular ultrasound follow-up, these stents disappeared from the vessel in about three years.

In 2009, a clinical trial, with limited patient enrollment, was conducted to explore the effect of bioabsorbable everolimus-eluting coronary stents on patients with coronary artery atherosclerosis [123]. At 2 year follow-up, some struts had disappeared, and the vessels in the area of the stent had regained normal vasomotor function.

When suitable biodegradable materials became available, in addition to metallic stents, this material was explored for use as scaffolds for tissue engineering and vascular grafts. What was the role of heparin in this fast growing field?

Bioengineered tissue is usually composed of a supporting scaffold and different cellular elements of the interested organ. In tissue engineered vascular grafts, the scaffolds are often made of either a segment of decellularized blood vessel or a tubular structure made from biodegradable materials. The seeding cells could be endothelial cells, smooth muscle cells or progenitor cells from either circulating blood or bone marrow. In a recent animal study, Zhou et al used decellularized small vessels as scaffolds for vascular grafts [130]. Before seeding the cultured bone marrow mesenchymal cells, the scaffolds were treated with heparin. The results confirmed heparin's ability to enhance cell adhesion, and proliferation. In contrast, in Yu's study, segments of PLLA and polycaprolactone (PCL) microfiber-made bioabsorbable tubules were used as a scaffold for grafting [131]. Three different types of grafts were used; grafts with polymer alone, grafts coated with heparin, and grafts coated with both heparin and stromal cell-derived factor-1α (SCF-1 α). The group with both heparin and SCF-1 α had recruited significant numbers of endothelial cells on the grafted vessel wall in the initial phase, and demonstrated a better endothelial lining and luminal patency in the later phase.

The above are just few examples of heparin's effects on cardiovascular interventional management in patients with atherosclerosis. Heparin is a mandatory antithrombotic agent for patients undergoing the PTCA procedure. Heparin had also been used in different trials in bare metal stents, and drug eluting metal stents. The use of heparin in the development of bioabsorbable materials and their application in temporary stents and vessel tissue engineering has added a new use for this compound in vascular medicine.

Conclusion

Although the drug heparin has been used in cardiovascular medicine for almost eighty years it continues to have unlimited value. Scientists and clinicians have focused on the anticoagulant properties of heparin to prevent thrombosis. New anticoagulant drugs, such as specific Xa and IIa inhibitors, are current candidates to replace heparin's use as an anticoagulant but many other attributes of the diverse heparin molecule make it useful in prevention of thrombosis and in other applications in cardiovascular medicine. In the present article we discuss the interaction of heparin with the vessel wall and the importance of this interaction in heparin's antithrombotic activity and its potential to prevent and treat atherosclerosis. The interaction of heparin with the vasculature, may also prevent the cardiovascular complications associated with diabetes including protection of the glomerular membrane in the kidney [132]. Heparin may also prolong survival in cancer patients by mechanisms other than that associated with coagulation [133]. Thus further study on the interaction of heparin with the endothelium but also leukocytes and smooth muscle cells are required to fully harness the potential of heparin and derived compounds.

References

[1] Esko, J. D.; Kimata, K.; Lindahl, U. (2009). Proteoglycans and Sulfated Glycosaminoglycans. In: A. Varki, R. D. Cummings, J. D. Esko, H. H. Freeze, P. Stanley, C. Bertozzi, G. W. art, M. E. tzler (Eds.), *Essentials of Glycobiology* (2nd, 1-39). New York: Cold Spring Harbor Laboratory Press.

[2] Abrink, M.; Grujic, M.; Pejler, G. (2004). Serglycin is essential for maturation of mast cell secretory granule. *J Biol Chem, 279,* 40897-40905.

[3] Linhardt, R. J. & Loganathan, D. (1990). Heparin, Heparinoids and Heparin Oligosaccharides: Structure and Biological Activities. In:

G.Gebelein (Eds.), *Biomimetic Polymers* (135-173). New York: Plenum Press.

[4] Fareed, J.; Ma, Q.; Florian, M.; Maddineni, J.; Iqbal, O.; Hoppensteadt, D. A.; Bick, R. (2003). Unfractionated and low-molecular-weight heparins, basic mechansim of action and pharmacology. *Seminars in Cardiothoracic and Vascular Anaesthesia, 7,* 357-377.

[5] Frydman, A. M.; Bara, L.; LeRous, Y.; Moler, M.; Chaulic, F. (1988). The antithrombotic activity and pharmacokinetics of Enoxaparine, a low molecular weight heparin, in humans given a single subcutaneous dose of 20 to 80 mg. *Journal of Clinical Pharmacology, 28,* 609-618.

[6] Palm, M.; Wu, H.; Mattsson, C.; Ansari, A. (1990). Pharmacokinetic properties of size-homogenous heparin oligosaccharides. *Thrombosis Research, 59,* 799-805.

[7] Xu, Y.; Masuko, S.; Takieddin, M.; Xu, H.; Liu, R.; Jing, J.; Mousa, S. A.; Linhardt, R. J.; Liu, J. (2011). Chemoenzymatic synthesis of homogeneous ultralow molecular weight heparins. *Science, 334,* 498-501.

[8] Varki, A. (2002). Six Blind men and the elephant-the many faces of heparan sulfate. *PNAS, 99,* 543-545.

[9] Sasisekharan, R.; Shriver, Z.; Venkataraman, G.; Narayanasami, U. (2002). Roles of heparan-sulphate glycosaminoglycans in cancer. *Nat Rev Cancer, 2,* 521-528.

[10] Linhardt RJ. (2003). Heparin: structure and activity. *J Med Chem, 46,* 2551-2564.

[11] Hileman, R.; Fromm, J.; Wieler, J.; Linchardt, R. (1998). Glycosaminoglycan-protein interations:definition of consensus sites in glycosaminoglycan binding proteins. *Bioessays, 20,* 156-167.

[12] Rosenberg, R. D.; Shworak, N. W.; Liu, J.; Schwartz, J. J.; Zhang, L. (1997). Heparan sulfate proteoglycans of the cardiovascular system. Specific structures emerge but how is synthesis regulated? *J Clin Invest, 99,* 2062-2070.

[13] Kolset, S. & Salmivirta, M. (1999). Cell surface heparan sulfate proteoglycans and lipoprotein metabolism. *Cellular and Molecular Life Sciences, 56,* 857-870.

[14] Florian, J. A.; Kosky, J. R.; Ainslie, K.; Pang, Z.; Dull, R. O.; Tarbell, J. M. (2003). Heparan sulfate proteoglycan is a mechanosensor on endothelial cells. *Circulation Research, 93,* e136-e142.

[15] Mahley, R. W. J. Z. S. (1999). Remnant lipoprotein metabolism: key pathways involving cell-surface heparan sulfate proteoglycans and apolipoprotein E. *J Lipid Res, 40,* 1-16.

[16] Bjork, I.; Olson, S. T.; Shore, J. D. (1989). Molecular mechanisms of the accelerating effect of heparin on the reactions between antithrombin and clotting proteinases. In: D. A. Lane & U. Lindahl (Eds.), *Heparin: Chemical and Biological Properties Clinical Applications* (1, 229-255). Boca Raton,Florida: CRC Press,Inc.

[17] Ludwig-Baxter, K. G.; Rej, R. N.; Perlin, A. S.; Neville, G. A. (1991). A novel method for differentiating dextran sulfate from related sulfated polysaccharides. *Journal of Pharmaceutical Sciences, 80,7,* 655-660.

[18] Harenberg, J.; Haaf, B.; Schafer, M.; Dempfle, C.; Stehle, G.; Heene, D. (1993). Anti-factor Xa determination in blood: a new method for controlling heparin therapy. *Seminars in Thrombosis and Hemostasis, 19, Suppl.1.,* 79-85.

[19] Morris, T. (2003). Heparin and low molecular weight heparin: background and pharmacology. *Clin Chest Med, 24,* 39-47.

[20] Bara, L.; Planes, A.; Samama, M. M. (1999). Occurence of thrombosis and haemorrhage, relationship with anti-Xa, anti-IIa activities, and D-dimer plasma levels in patients receiving low molecular weight heparin, enoxaparin or tinzaparin, to prevent deep vein thrombosis after hip surgery. *British Journal of Haematology, 104,* 230-240.

[21] Hoppensteadt, D.; Walenga, J.; Fasanella, A.; Jeske, W.; Fareed, J. (1995). TFPI antigen levels in normal human volunteers after intravenous and subcutaneous administration of unfractionated and a low molecular weight heparin. *Thrombosis Research, 77,2,* 175-185.

[22] Dahm, A.; Van, H., V; Bendz, B.; Rosendaal, F.; Bertina, R. M.; Sandset, P. M. (2003). Low levels of tissue factor pathway inhibitor (TFPI) increase the risk of venous thrombosis. *Blood, 101,* 4387-4392.

[23] Aird, W. C. (2007). Phenotypic heterogeneity of the endothelium: I. Structure, function, and mechanisms. *Circ Res, 100,* 158-173.

[24] Hoffmann, J.; Haendeler, J.; Aicher, A.; Rossig, L.; Vasa, M.; Zeiher, A. M.; Dimmeler, S. (2001). Aging enhances the sensitivity of endothelial cells toward apoptotic stimuli: important role of nitric oxide. *Circulation Research, 89,* 709-715.

[25] Mehta, D. & Malik, A. B. (2006). Signaling mechanisms regulating endothelial permeability. *Physiol Rev, 86,* 279-367.

[26] Kofler, S.; Nickel, T.; Weis, M. (2005). Role of cytokines in cardiovascular diseases: a focus on endothelial responses to inflammation. *Clin Sci (Lond), 108,* 205-213.

[27] Reitsma, S.; Slaaf, D. W.; Vink, H.; van Zandvoort, M. A.; oude Egbrink, M. G. (2007). The endothelial glycocalyx: composition, functions, and visualization. *Pflugers Arch, 454,* 345-359.

[28] Lennon, F. E. & Singleton, P. A. (2011). Hyaluronan regulation of vascular integrity. *Am J Cardiovasc Dis, 1,* 200-213.

[29] Gambaro, G. & Baggio, B. (1992). Role of glycosaminoglycans in diabetic nephropathy. *Acta Diabetol, 29,* 149-155.

[30] Kanwar, Y. S.; Linker, A.; Farquhar, M. G. (1980). Increased permeability of the glomerular basement membrane to ferritin aftr removal of glycosaminoglycans (heparan sulphate) by enzyme digestion. *Journal of Cell Biology, 86,* 688-693.

[31] Kanwar, Y. S.; Rosenzweig, L. J.; Linker, A.; Jakubowski, M. L. (1983). Decreased de novo synthesis of glomerular proteoglycans in diabetes: Biochemical and autoradiographic evidence. *Proceedings of the National Academy of Sciences of the United States of America, 80,* 2272-2275.

[32] Ilse Raats, C. J.; van den Born, J.; Berden, J. H. M. (2000). Glomerular heparan sulfate alterations: Mechanisms and relevance for proteinuria. *Kidney International, 57,* 385-400.

[33] Owens, G. K. (1995). Regulation of differentiation of vascular smooth muscle cells. *Physiol. Rev, 75,* 487-517.

[34] Munoz, E. M. & Linhardt, R. J. (2004). Heparin-binding domains in vascular biology. *Arteriosclerosis Thrombosis and Vascular Biology, 24,* 1549-1557.

[35] Hiebert, L. M. & McDuffie, N. M. (1989). The intracellular uptake and protracted release of exogenous heparins by cultured endothelial cells. *Artery, 16,* 208-222.

[36] Glimelius, B.; Busch, C.; Hook, M. (1978). Binding of heparin on the surface of cultured human endothelial cells. *Thrombosis Research, 12,* 773-782.

[37] Barzu, T.; Molho, P.; Toblelem, G.; Petitou, M.; Caen, J. P. (1984). Binding of Heparin and low molecular weight heparin fragments to human vascular endothelial cells in culture. *Nouvelle Revue Francaise d'Hematologie, 26,* 243-247.

[38] Barzu, T.; Molho, P.; Tobelem, G.; Petitou, M.; Caen, J. (1985). Binding and endocytosis of heparin by human endothelial cells in culture. *Biochimica et Biophysica Acta, 845,* 196-203.

[39] Barzu, T.; Van Rijn, J. L. M. L.; Petitou, M.; Molho, P.; Tobelem, G.; Caen, J. P. (1986). Endothelial binding sites for heparin. *Biochemistry Journal, 238,* 847-854.

[40] van Rijn, J. L. M. L.; Trillou, M.; Mardiguian, J.; Tobelem, G.; Caen, J. (1987). Selective binding of heparins to human endothelial cells. Implications for pharmacokinetics. *Thrombosis Research, 45,* 211-222.

[41] Vannucchi, S.; Pasquali, F.; Chiarugi, V.; Ruggiero, M. (1986). Internalization and metabolism of endogenous heparin by cultured endothelial cells. *Biochemical and Biophysical Research Communications, 140,* 294-301.

[42] Vannucchi, S.; Pasquali, F.; Porciatti, F.; Chiarugi, V.; Magnelli, L.; Bianchini, P. (1988). Binding, internalization and degradation of heparin and heparin fragments by cultured endothelial cells. *Thrombosis Research, 49,* 373-383.

[43] Hiebert, L. M. & Jaques, L. B. (1976). Heparin uptake on endothelium. *Artery, 2,1,* 26-37.

[44] Hiebert, L. M. & Jaques, L. B. (1976). The observation of heparin on endothelium after injection. *Thrombosis Research, 8,* 195-204.

[45] Hiebert, L. M. (1979). Heparin and Endothelium. In: N. M. McDuffie (Eds.), *Heparin, Structure, Cellular Functions and Clinical Applications* (289-297). New York: Academic Press.

[46] Jaques, L. B.; Hiebert, L. M.; Wice, S. M. (1991). Evidence from endothelium of gastric absorption of heparin and of dextran sulfates 8000. *Journal of Laboratory and Clinical Medicine, 117,2.,* 122-130.

[47] Hiebert, L. M.; Wice, S. M.; McDuffie, N. M.; Jaques, L. B. (1993). The heparin target organ - the endothelium. Studies in a rat model. *The Quarterly Journal of Medicine, 86,* 341-348.

[48] Dawes, J. & Pepper, D. (1992). Human vascular endothelial cells catabolise exogenous glycosaminoglycans by a novel route. *Thrombosis and Haemostasis, 67,4,* 468-472.

[49] Barzu, T.; van Rijn, J. L. M. L.; Petitou, M.; Tobelem, G.; Caen, J. P. (1987). Heparin degradation in endothelial cells. *Thrombosis Research, 47,* 601-609.

[50] Hiebert, L. M. & McDuffie, N. M. (1990). The internalization and release of heparins by cultured endothelial cells: The process is cell

source, heparin source, time and concentration dependent. *Artery, 17,* 107-118.

[51] Folkman, J.; Langer, R.; Linhardt, R. J.; Haudenschild, C.; Taylor, S. (1983). Angiogenesis inhibition and tumor regression caused by heparin or a heparin fragment in the presence of cortisone. *Science, 221,* 719-725.

[52] Folkman, J.; Weisz, P. B.; Joullie, M. M.; Li, W. W.; Ewing, W. R. (1989). Control of angiogenesis with synthetic heparin substitutes. *Science, 243,* 1490-1493.

[53] Norrby, K. (1993). Heparin and angiogenesis:A low-molecular weight fraction inhibits and a high-molecular weight fraction stimulates angiogenesis systemically. *Haemostasis, 23,Suppl,* 141-149.

[54] Stins, M. F.; Maxfield, F. R.; Goldberg, I. J. (1992). Polarized binding of lipoprotein lipase to endothelial cells. *Arteriosclerosis Thrombosis and Vascular Biology, 12,* 1437-1446.

[55] Kojima, H.; Omoto, Y.; Hidaka, H.; Aoki, T.; Nakamura, T.; Kawabata, T.; Konaka, K.; Kashiwagi, A.; Kikkawa, R.; Shigeta, Y. (1992). Increased plasma post-heparin diamine oxidase activity and plant sterol levels in streptozotocin diabetic rat. *Biochemical and Biophysical Research Communications, 186,1,* 398-404.

[56] Oyanagui, Y. & Sato, S. (1990). Heparin, a potent releasing agent of extracellular superoxide dismutase (EC-SOD C), suppersses ischaemic paw oedema in mice. *Free Radical Research Communications, 9,* 87-99.

[57] Yasuba, H.; Chihara, J.; Kino, T.; Satake, N.; Oshima, S. (1991). Increased releasability of platelet products and reduced heparin- induced platelet factor 4 release from endothelial cells in bronchial asthma. *Journal of Lipid Mediators, 4,* 5-22.

[58] Hiebert, L. M. & Liu, J. (1990). Heparin protects cultured endothelial cells from damage by toxic oxygen metabolites. *Atherosclerosis, 83,* 47-51.

[59] Hiebert, L. M. & Liu, J. (1991). Protective action of polyelectrolytes on endothelium. *Seminars in Thrombosis and Hemostasis, 17(Supp 1),* 42-46.

[60] Black, S. C.; Gralinski, M. R.; Friedrichs, G. S.; Kilgore, K. S.; Driscoll, E. M.; Lucchesi, B. R. (1995). Cardioprotective effects of heparin or N-acetylheparin in an in vivo model of myocardial ischaemic and reperfusion injury. *Cardiovascular Research, 29,* 629-636.

[61] Han, J.; Mandal, A. K.; Hiebert, L. M. (2005). Endothelial cell injury by high glucose and heparanase is prevented by insulin, heparin and basic

fibroblast growth factor. *Cardiovascular Diabetology, 4,* 12-Available from URL: http://www.cardiab.com/content/4/1/12.

[62] Han, J.; Zhang, F.; Xie, J.; Linhardt, R. J.; Hiebert, L. M. (2009). Changes in cultured endothelial cell glycosaminoglycans under hyperglycemic conditions and the effect of insulin and heparin. *Cardiovascular Diabetology, 8,* 46-

[63] Fairman, R. P.; Sessler, C. N.; Bierman, M.; Glauser, F. L. (1987). Protamine sulfate causes pulmonary hypertension and edema in isolated rat lungs. *Journal of Applied Physiology, 62,* 1363-1367.

[64] Nader, N. B.; Toma, L.; Pinhal, M. A. S.; Buonassisi, V.; Colburn, P.; Dietrich, C. P. (1991). Effect of heparin and dextran sulfate on the synthesis and structure of heparan sulfate from cultured endothelial cells. *Seminars in Thrombosis and Hemostasis, 17,* 47-56.

[65] Pinhal, M. A.; Walenga, J. M.; Jeske, W.; Hoppensteadt, D.; Dietrich, C. P.; Fareed, J.; Nader, H. B. (1994). Antithrombotic agents stimulate the synthesis and modify the sulfation pattern of a heparan sulfate proteoglycan from endothelial cells. *Thrombosis Research, 74,* 143-153.

[66] Mandal, A. K.; Lyden, T.; Saklayen, M. G. (1995). Heparin lowers blood pressure:Biological and clinical perspectives. *Kidney International, 47,* 1017-1022.

[67] Young, E. (2008). The anti-inflammatory effects of heparin and related compounds. *Thrombosis Research, 122,* 743-752.

[68] Wang, L.; Fuster, M.; Sriramarao, P.; Esko, J. D. (2005). Endothelial heparan sulfate deficiency impairs L-selectin- and chemokine-mediated neutrophil trafficking during inflammatory responses. *Nature Immunology, 6,* 902-910.

[69] Peter, K.; Schwarz, M.; Conradt, C.; Nordt, T.; Moser, M.; Kubler, W.; Bode, C. (1999). Heparin inhibits ligand binding to the leukocyte integrin Mac-1 (CD11b/CD18). *Circulation, 100,* 1533-1539.

[70] Brown, R. A.; Lever, R.; Jones, N. A.; Page, C. P. (2003). Effects of heparin and related molecules upon neutrophil aggregation and elastase release in vitro. *British Journal of Clinical Pharmacology, 139,* 845-853.

[71] Manduteanu, I.; Voinea, M.; Antohe, F.; Dragomir, E.; Capraru, M.; Radulescu, L.; Simionescu, M. (2003). Effect of enoxaparin on high glucose-induced activation of endothelial cells. *European Journal of Pharmacology, 477,* 269-276.

[72] Hecht, I.; Hershkoviz, R.; Shivtiel, S.; Lapidot, T.; Cohen, I. R.; Lider, O.; Cahalon, L. (2004). Heparin-disaccharide affects T cells: inhibition

of NF-kappaB activation, cell migration, and modulation of intracellular signaling. *J. Leukoc. Biol., 75,* 1139-1146.

[73] Clowes, A. W. & Karnovsky, M. J. (1977). Supression by heparin of smooth muscle cell proliferation in injured arteries. *Nature, 265,* 625-626.

[74] Pukac, L. A.; Castellot, J. J.; Wright, T.; Caleb, B. L.; Karnovsky, M. J. (1990). Heparin inhibits c-fos and c-myc RNA expression in vascular smooth muscle cells. *Cell Regulation, 1,5,* 435-443.

[75] Pukac, L. A.; Ottlinger, M. E.; Karnovsky, M. J. (1992). Heparin suppresses specific 2nd messenger pathways for protooncogene expression in rat vascular smooth muscle cells. *Journal of Biological Chemistry, 267,6,* 3707-3711.

[76] Fager, G.; Camejo, G.; Bondjers, G. (1995). Heparin-like glycosaminoglycans influence growth and phenotype of human arterial smooth muscle cells in vitro. II.The platelet derived factor A-chain contains a sequence that specifically binds heparin. *In Vitro Cellular and Developmental Biology, 28A,* 176-180.

[77] Hoover, R. L.; Rosenberg, R.; Haering, W.; Karnovsky, M. J. (1980). Inhibition of rat arterial smooth muscle cell proliferation by heparin. II. In vitro studies. *Circ. Res., 47,* 578-583.

[78] Castellot, J. J.; Addonizio, M.; Rosenberg, R.; Karnovsky, M. J. (1981). Cultured endothelial cells produce a heparin like inhibitor of smooth muscle growth. *Journal of Cell Biology, 90,* 372-380.

[79] Fritze, L. M. S.; Reilly, C. F.; Rosenberg, R. D. (1985). Antiproliferative heparan sulfate species produced by post confluent smooth muscle cells. *Journal of Cell Biology, 100,* 1041-1049.

[80] Kilfeather, S. A.; Tagoe, S.; Perez, A. C.; Okona-Mensa, K.; Matin, R.; Page, C. P. (1995). Inhibition of serum-induced proliferation of bovine tracheal smooth muscle cells in culture by heparin and related glycosaminoglycans. *Br. J. Pharmacol., 114,* 1442-1446.

[81] Benitz, W. E.; Kelley, R. T.; Anderson, C. M.; Lorant, D. E.; Bernfield, M. (1990). Endothelial heparan sulfate proteoglycan. I. Inhibitory effects on smooth muscle cell proliferation. *Am. J. Respir. Cell Mol. Biol., 2,* 13-24.

[82] Bigelow, W. G. (1990). Mysterious heparin, the key to open heart surgery. *1,* 1-205.

[83] Araki, H.; Muramoto, J.; Nishi, K.; Jougasaki, M.; Inoue, M.; Demichele, M. A. A. (1992). Heparin adheres to the damaged arterial

wall and inhibits its thrombogenicity. *Circulation Research, 71,3,* 577-884.

[84] Arbit, E.; Goldberg, M.; Gomez-Orellana, I.; Majuru, S. (2006). Oral heparin: status review. *Thromb. J., 4,* 6-

[85] Dryjski, M.; Schneider, D. E.; Mojaverian, P.; Kuo, B.; Bjornsson, T. D. (1989). Investigations on plasma activity of low molecular weight heparin after intravenous and oral administrations. *British Journal of Clinical Pharmacology, 28,* 188-192.

[86] Hiebert, L. M.; Wice, S. M.; Jaques, L. B. (1996). Antithrombotic activity of oral unfractionated heparin. *Journal of Cardiovascular Pharmacology, 28,* 26-29.

[87] Hiebert, L. M. (2002). Oral heparins. *Clinical Laboratory, 48,* 111-116.

[88] Hiebert, L. M.; Ping, T.; Wice, S. M. (2000). Antithrombotic activity of orally administered low molecular weight heparin (logiparin) in a rat model. *Haemostasis, 30,* 196-203.

[89] Hiebert, L. M.; Wice, S. M.; Ping, T.; Herr, D.; Laux, V. (2001). Antithrombotic efficacy in a rat model of the low molecular weight heparin, reviparin sodium, administered by the oral route. *Thrombosis and Haemostasis, 85,* 114-118.

[90] Pinel, C.; Wice, S. M.; Hiebert, L. M. (2004). Orally administered heparins prevent arterial thrombosis in a rat model. *Thrombosis and Haemostasis, 91,* 919-926.

[91] Hiebert, L. M. (2004). Evidence that orally administered heparins are absorbed. In: J. Vossoughi, J. Fareed, S. A. Mousa, J. W. Karanian (Eds.), *Thrombosis Research and Treatment. Bench to Bedside* (1, 553-563). Washington DC: Medical and Engineering Publishers, Inc.

[92] Hiebert, L. M.; Wice, S. M.; Ping, T.; Hileman, R. E.; Capila, I.; Linhardt, R. J. (2000). Tissue distribution and antithrombotic activity of unlabeled or ^{14}C-labeled porcine intestinal mucosal heparin following administration to rats by the oral route. *Canadian Journal of Physiology and Pharmacology, 78,* 307-320.

[93] Hiebert, L. M.; Ping, T.; Wice, S. M. (2011). Repeated doses of oral and subcutaneous heparins have similar antithrombotic effects in a rat carotid arterial model of thrombosis. *Journal of Cardiovascular Pharmacology and Therapeutics,*

[94] Daniels, B.; Linhardt, R. J.; Zhang, F.; Mao, W.; Wice, S. M.; Hiebert, L. M. (2006). In vivo antithrombotic synergy of oral heparin and arginine: endothelial thromboresistance without changes in coagulation parameters. *Thrombosis and Haemostasis, 95,* 865-872.

[95] Engelberg, H. (1980). Heparin and atherosclerosis. A review of old and recent findings. *American Heart Journal, 99(3),* 359-372.

[96] Engelberg, H. (1990). Heparin and the Prevention of Atherosclerosis: Basic Research and Clinical Application.

[97] Engelberg, H. (1996). Actions of heparin in the atherosclerotic process. *Pharmacological Reviews, 48,* 327-352.

[98] Murata, K.; Murata, A.; Yoshida, K. (1997). Heparan sulfate isomers in cerebral arteries of Japanese women with aging and with atherosclerosis--heparitinase and high-performance liquid chromatography determinations. *Atherosclerosis, 132,* 9-17.

[99] Nader, H. B.; Buonassisi, V.; Colburn, P.; Dietrich, C. P. (1989). Heparin stimulates the synthesis and modifies the sulfation pattern of heparan sulfate proteoglycan from endothelial cells. *Journal of Cellular Physiology, 140,* 305-310.

[100] Light, J. T.; Bellan, J. A.; Roberts, M. P.; Force, S. D.; Chen, I. L.; Kerstein, M. D.; Kadowitz, P. J.; McNamara, D. B. (1993). Heparin treatment enhances the recovery of neoendothelial acetylcholine-induced vascular relaxation after balloon catheter injury in the rabbit aorta. *Circulation, 88,* II413-II419.

[101] Hunt, D. (2004). Low molecular weight heparin and atherosclerosis. *Curr Atheroscler Rep, 6,* 140-147.

[102] Wang, Q. S.; Chen, C.; Chen, X. Y.; Han, J. H.; Soo, Y.; Leung, T. W.; Mok, V.; Wong, K. S. (2012). Low-molecular-weight heparin versus aspirin for acute ischemic stroke with large artery occlusive disease: subgroup analyses from the Fraxiparin in Stroke Study for the treatment of ischemic stroke (FISS-tris) study. *Stroke, 43,* 346-349.

[103] Nobuyoshi, M.; Kimura, T.; Ohishi, H.; Horiuchi, H.; Nosaka, H.; Hamasaki, N.; Yokoi, H.; Kim, K. (1991). Restenosis after percutaneous transluminal coronary angioplasty: pathologic observations in 20 patients. *J. Am. Coll. Cardiol., 17,* 433-439.

[104] Leimgruber, P. P.; Roubin, G. S.; Hollman, J.; Cotsonis, G. A.; Meier, B.; Douglas, J. S.; King, S. B., Jr.; Gruentzig, A. R. (1986). Restenosis after successful coronary angioplasty in patients with single-vessel disease. *Circulation, 73,* 710-717.

[105] Gruentzig A. (1978). Transluminal dilatation of coronary-artery stenosis (letter). *Lancet, 311,* 263-263.

[106] Gruentzig, A. R.; King, S. B., III; Schlumpf, M.; Siegenthaler, W. (1987). Long-term follow-up after percutaneous transluminal coronary

angioplasty. The early Zurich experience. *N. Engl. J. Med., 316,* 1127-1132.

[107] Fischman, D. L.; Leon, M. B.; Baim, D. S.; Schatz, R. A.; Savage, M. P.; Penn, I.; Detre, K.; Veltri, L.; Ricci, D.; Nobuyoshi, M.; . (1994). A randomized comparison of coronary-stent placement and balloon angioplasty in the treatment of coronary artery disease. Stent Restenosis Study Investigators. *N. Engl. J. Med., 331,* 496-501.

[108] Liistro, F.; Stankovic, G.; Di, M. C.; Takagi, T.; Chieffo, A.; Moshiri, S.; Montorfano, M.; Carlino, M.; Briguori, C.; Pagnotta, P.; Albiero, R.; Corvaja, N.; Colombo, A. (2002). First clinical experience with a paclitaxel derivate-eluting polymer stent system implantation for in-stent restenosis: immediate and long-term clinical and angiographic outcome. *Circulation, 105,* 1883-1886.

[109] Morice, M. C.; Serruys, P. W.; Sousa, J. E.; Fajadet, J.; Ban, H. E.; Perin, M.; Colombo, A.; Schuler, G.; Barragan, P.; Guagliumi, G.; Molnar, F.; Falotico, R. (2002). A randomized comparison of a sirolimus-eluting stent with a standard stent for coronary revascularization. *N. Engl. J. Med., 346,* 1773-1780.

[110] Stettler, C.; Wandel, S.; Allemann, S.; Kastrati, A.; Morice, M. C.; Schomig, A.; Pfisterer, M. E.; Stone, G. W.; Leon, M. B.; de Lezo, J. S.; Goy, J. J.; Park, S. J.; Sabate, M.; Suttorp, M. J.; Kelbaek, H.; Spaulding, C.; Menichelli, M.; Vermeersch, P.; Dirksen, M. T.; Cervinka, P.; Petronio, A. S.; Nordmann, A. J.; Diem, P.; Meier, B.; Zwahlen, M.; Reichenbach, S.; Trelle, S.; Windecker, S.; Juni, P. (2007). Outcomes associated with drug-eluting and bare-metal stents: a collaborative network meta-analysis. *Lancet, 370,* 937-948.

[111] Serruys, P. W.; Onuma, Y.; Ormiston, J. A.; de, B. B.; Regar, E.; Dudek, D.; Thuesen, L.; Smits, P. C.; Chevalier, B.; McClean, D.; Koolen, J.; Windecker, S.; Whitbourn, R.; Meredith, I.; Dorange, C.; Veldhof, S.; Miquel-Hebert, K.; Rapoza, R.; Garcia-Garcia, H. M. (2010). Evaluation of the second generation of a bioresorbable everolimus drug-eluting vascular scaffold for treatment of de novo coronary artery stenosis: six-month clinical and imaging outcomes. *Circulation, 122,* 2301-2312.

[112] Raber, L.; Kelbaek, H.; Ostojic, M.; Baumbach, A.; Heg, D.; Tuller, D.; von, B. C.; Roffi, M.; Moschovitis, A.; Khattab, A. A.; Wenaweser, P.; Bonvini, R.; Pedrazzini, G.; Kornowski, R.; Weber, K.; Trelle, S.; Luscher, T. F.; Taniwaki, M.; Matter, C. M.; Meier, B.; Juni, P.; Windecker, S. (2012). Effect of biolimus-eluting stents with biodegradable polymer vs bare-metal stents on cardiovascular events

among patients with acute myocardial infarction: the COMFORTABLE AMI randomized trial. *Journal of the American Medical Association, 308,* 777-787.

[113] Scheller, B.; Hehrlein, C.; Bocksch, W.; Rutsch, W.; Haghi, D.; Dietz, U.; Bohm, M.; Speck, U. (2006). Treatment of coronary in-stent restenosis with a paclitaxel-coated balloon catheter. *N. Engl. J. Med., 355,* 2113-2124.

[114] Komatsu, R.; Ueda, M.; Naruko, T.; Kojima, A.; Becker, A. E. (1998). Neointimal tissue response at sites of coronary stenting in humans: macroscopic, histological, and immunohistochemical analyses. *Circulation, 98,* 224-233.

[115] Joner, M.; Finn, A. V.; Farb, A.; Mont, E. K.; Kolodgie, F. D.; Ladich, E.; Kutys, R.; Skorija, K.; Gold, H. K.; Virmani, R. (2006). Pathology of drug-eluting stents in humans: delayed healing and late thrombotic risk. *J. Am. Coll. Cardiol., 48,* 193-202.

[116] Guagliumi, G.; Sirbu, V.; Musumeci, G.; Gerber, R.; Biondi-Zoccai, G.; Ikejima, H.; Ladich, E.; Lortkipanidze, N.; Matiashvili, A.; Valsecchi, O.; Virmani, R.; Stone, G. W. (2012). Examination of the in vivo mechanisms of late drug-eluting stent thrombosis: findings from optical coherence tomography and intravascular ultrasound imaging. *JACC Cardiovasc. Interv., 5,* 12-20.

[117] Cook, S.; Wenaweser, P.; Togni, M.; Billinger, M.; Morger, C.; Seiler, C.; Vogel, R.; Hess, O.; Meier, B.; Windecker, S. (2007). Incomplete stent apposition and very late stent thrombosis after drug-eluting stent implantation. *Circulation, 115,* 2426-2434.

[118] Moreno, R.; Fernandez, C.; Hernandez, R.; Alfonso, F.; Angiolillo, D. J.; Sabate, M.; Escaned, J.; Banuelos, C.; Fernandez-Ortiz, A.; Macaya, C. (2005). Drug-eluting stent thrombosis: results from a pooled analysis including 10 randomized studies. *J. Am. Coll. Cardiol., 45,* 954-959.

[119] Cutlip, D. E.; Baim, D. S.; Ho, K. K.; Popma, J. J.; Lansky, A. J.; Cohen, D. J.; Carrozza, J. P., Jr.; Chauhan, M. S.; Rodriguez, O.; Kuntz, R. E. (2001). Stent thrombosis in the modern era: a pooled analysis of multicenter coronary stent clinical trials. *Circulation, 103,* 1967-1971.

[120] Virmani, R.; Guagliumi, G.; Farb, A.; Musumeci, G.; Grieco, N.; Motta, T.; Mihalcsik, L.; Tespili, M.; Valsecchi, O.; Kolodgie, F. D. (2004). Localized hypersensitivity and late coronary thrombosis secondary to a sirolimus-eluting stent: should we be cautious? *Circulation, 109,* 701-705.

[121] Ong, A. T.; van Domburg, R. T.; Aoki, J.; Sonnenschein, K.; Lemos, P. A.; Serruys, P. W. (2006). Sirolimus-eluting stents remain superior to bare-metal stents at two years: medium-term results from the Rapamycin-Eluting Stent Evaluated at Rotterdam Cardiology Hospital (RESEARCH) registry. *J. Am. Coll. Cardiol., 47,* 1356-1360.

[122] Ormiston, J. A.; Serruys, P. W.; Regar, E.; Dudek, D.; Thuesen, L.; Webster, M. W.; Onuma, Y.; Garcia-Garcia, H. M.; McGreevy, R.; Veldhof, S. (2008). A bioabsorbable everolimus-eluting coronary stent system for patients with single de-novo coronary artery lesions (ABSORB): a prospective open-label trial. *Lancet, 371,* 899-907.

[123] Serruys, P. W.; Ormiston, J. A.; Onuma, Y.; Regar, E.; Gonzalo, N.; Garcia-Garcia, H. M.; Nieman, K.; Bruining, N.; Dorange, C.; Miquel-Hebert, K.; Veldhof, S.; Webster, M.; Thuesen, L.; Dudek, D. (2009). A bioabsorbable everolimus-eluting coronary stent system (ABSORB): 2-year outcomes and results from multiple imaging methods. *Lancet, 373,* 897-910.

[124] Serruys, P. W.; Emanuelsson, H.; van der Giessen, W.; Lunn, A. C.; Kiemeney, F.; Macaya, C.; Rutsch, W.; Heyndrickx, G.; Suryapranata, H.; Legrand, V.; Goy, J. J.; Materne, P.; Bonnier, H.; Morice, M. C.; Fajadet, J.; Belardi, J.; Colombo, A.; Garcia, E.; Ruygrok, P.; de, J. P.; Morel, M. A. (1996). Heparin-coated Palmaz-Schatz stents in human coronary arteries. Early outcome of the Benestent-II Pilot Study. *Circulation, 93,* 412-422.

[125] Serruys, P. W.; van, H. B.; Bonnier, H.; Legrand, V.; Garcia, E.; Macaya, C.; Sousa, E.; van der Giessen, W.; Colombo, A.; Seabra-Gomes, R.; Kiemeneij, F.; Ruygrok, P.; Ormiston, J.; Emanuelsson, H.; Fajadet, J.; Haude, M.; Klugmann, S.; Morel, M. A. (1998). Randomised comparison of implantation of heparin-coated stents with balloon angioplasty in selected patients with coronary artery disease (Benestent II). *Lancet, 352,* 673-681.

[126] Vrolix, M. C.; Legrand, V. M.; Reiber, J. H.; Grollier, G.; Schalij, M. J.; Brunel, P.; Martinez-Elbal, L.; Gomez-Recio, M.; Bar, F. W.; Bertrand, M. E.; Colombo, A.; Brachman, J. (2000). Heparin-coated Wiktor stents in human coronary arteries (MENTOR trial). MENTOR Trial Investigators. *Am. J. Cardiol., 86,* 385-389.

[127] Wohrle, J.; Al-Khayer, E.; Grotzinger, U.; Schindler, C.; Kochs, M.; Hombach, V.; Hoher, M. (2001). Comparison of the heparin coated vs the uncoated Jostent--no influence on restenosis or clinical outcome. *Eur. Heart J., 22,* 1808-1816.

[128] Tamai, H.; Igaki, K.; Kyo, E.; Kosuga, K.; Kawashima, A.; Matsui, S.; Komori, H.; Tsuji, T.; Motohara, S.; Uehata, H. (2000). Initial and 6-month results of biodegradable poly-l-lactic acid coronary stents in humans. *Circulation, 102,* 399-404.

[129] Nishio, S.; Kosuga, K.; Igaki, K.; Okada, M.; Kyo, E.; Tsuji, T.; Takeuchi, E.; Inuzuka, Y.; Takeda, S.; Hata, T.; Takeuchi, Y.; Kawada, Y.; Harita, T.; Seki, J.; Akamatsu, S.; Hasegawa, S.; Bruining, N.; Brugaletta, S.; de, W. S.; Muramatsu, T.; Onuma, Y.; Serruys, P. W.; Ikeguchi, S. (2012). Long-Term (>10 Years) clinical outcomes of first-in-human biodegradable poly-l-lactic acid coronary stents: Igaki-Tamai stents. *Circulation, 125,* 2343-2353.

[130] Zhou, M.; Liu, Z.; Liu, C.; Jiang, X.; Wei, Z.; Qiao, W.; Ran, F.; Wang, W.; Qiao, T.; Liu, C. (2012). Tissue engineering of small-diameter vascular grafts by endothelial progenitor cells seeding heparin-coated decellularized scaffolds. *J. Biomed. Mater. Res. B Appl. Biomater., 100,* 111-120.

[131] Yu, J.; Wang, A.; Tang, Z.; Henry, J.; Li-Ping, L. B.; Zhu, Y.; Yuan, F.; Huang, F.; Li, S. (2012). The effect of stromal cell-derived factor-1alpha/heparin coating of biodegradable vascular grafts on the recruitment of both endothelial and smooth muscle progenitor cells for accelerated regeneration. *Biomaterials, 33,* 8062-8074.

[132] Gambaro, G.; Kinalska, I.; Oksa, A.; Pont'usch, P.; Hertlova, M.; Olsovsky, J.; Manitius, J.; Fedele, D.; Czekalski, S.; Perusicova, J.; Skrl, J.; Taton, J.; Grezeszczak, W.; Crepaldi, G. (2002). Oral sulodexide reduces albuminuria in microalbuminuric and macroalbuminuric type 1 and type 2 diabetic patieints: the Di.N.A.S. randomized trial. *Journal of the American Society of Nephrology, 13,* 1615-1625.

[133] Aki, E. A. & Schünemann, H. J. (2012). Routine Heparin for Patients with Cancer? One Answer, More Questions. *New England Journal of Medicine, 366,* 661-662.

In: Heparin
Editor: Nicole B. Wilkinson

ISBN: 978-1-63117-624-1

Chapter IV

Intracellular Transport of Heparin-Binding EGF-Like Growth Factor (HB-EGF) and the Possibility of Targeted Drug Delivery to Distinct Intracellular Compartments

Miki Hieda
Graduate School of Medicine and Health Science,
Osaka University, Osaka, Japan

Abstract

Heparin-binding epidermal growth factor (EGF)-like growth factor (HB-EGF), a heparin-interacting protein, is synthesized as a type I transmembrane protein (proHB-EGF) in the ER, transported through the exocytic pathway, and expressed on the cell surface. Subsequently, proHB-EGF or a cleaved form, the carboxyl-terminal fragment of HB-EGF (HB-EGF-CTF), undergoes endocytosis and retrograde transport to several intracellular destinations including the Golgi, ER, lysosome, and inner nuclear membrane (INM).

Because they are internalized by endocytosis, cell-surface receptors and ligands can be used for drug delivery. At steady state, most endocytosed proteins are returned to the plasma membrane via endosomal recycling pathways; proteins that are not recycled are transported to distinct destinations. Well-defined membranes surround organelles, emphasizing the significance of the transport pathways that lead to distinct destinations. Thus, the choice of appropriate targets that are promptly transported to specific intracellular compartments is crucial for drug delivery. Here, I describe the intracellular transport of HB-EGF, focusing on retrograde transport pathways, and discuss the possibilities for exploiting HB-EGF transport in future drug-delivery systems.

Keywords: HB-EGF, intracellular trafficking, membrane trafficking, inner nuclear membrane, drug delivery

Abbreviations

EGF	epidermal growth factor
HB-EGF	heparin-binding EGF-like growth factor
EGFR	EGF receptor
CTF	carboxy-terminal fragment; nuclear envelope
INM	inner nuclear membrane
ONM	outer nuclear membrane

I. Intracellular Trafficking of HB-EGF

In 1990, a novel heparin-binding growth factor was identified in conditioned media of cultured peripheral blood mononuclear cells [1]. Shortly thereafter, this activity was purified and termed heparin-binding EGF-like growth factor, HB-EGF [2, 3]. HB-EGF belongs to the EGF-like growth factor family, which comprises seven members: EGF, amphiregulin, epiregulin, TGF-α, betacellulin, epigen, and HB-EGF (Figure 1). These molecules interact with and activate EGFR receptor (EGFR). HB-EGF is expressed in multiple tissues and participates in a variety of normal and aberrant processes including tumor growth; its structure and functions have been described elsewhere [4, 5]. Most cell-surface receptors are internalized through specific endocytic processes. Some of these pathways involve retrograde transport, by which proteins and lipids are transported from the plasma membrane to the

Golgi, ER, and even the inner nuclear membrane (INM) [6-8]. HB-EGF and another EGF-like growth factor, amphiregulin, both undergo intracellular transport from the plasma membrane to the INM [9-11], and are thus among the few plasma membrane proteins that have been demonstrated to be targeted to the INM (see below).

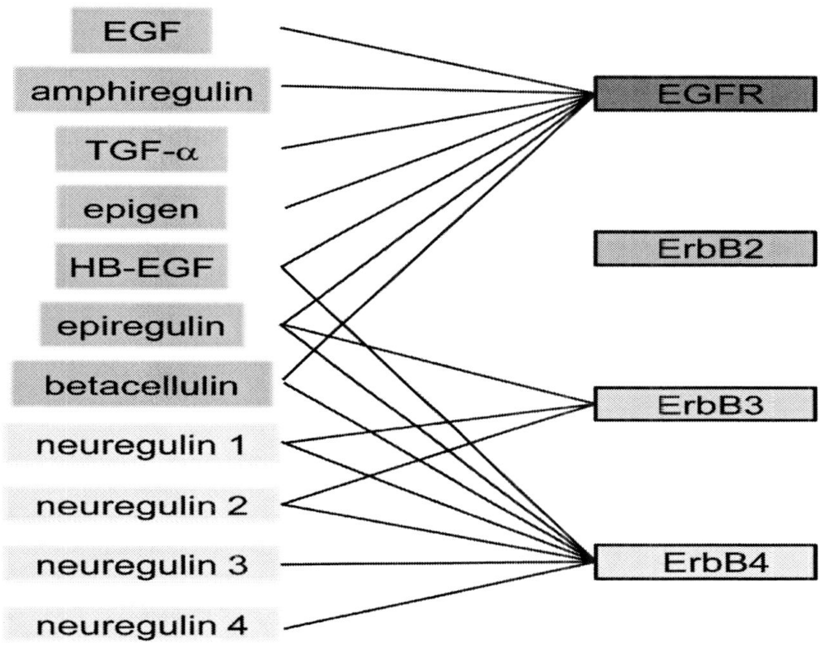

Figure 1. Proteins of the EGF receptor family and their ligands including both the EGF family and neuregulin family. EGF family members are type I transmembrane proteins that share a conserved EGF-like growth factor domain. The EGFR family comprises four structurally related receptor tyrosine kinases, EGFR (ErbB1, HER1), ErbB2 (HER2), ErbB3 (HER3), and ErbB4 (HER4), which form heterodimer. Neuregulin family proteins do not interact with EGFR, but interacts with ErbB4. It should be noted that the extracellular portions of HB-EGF and amphiregulin contain a heparin binding domain.

HB-EGF is synthesized at ER-bound ribosomes and expressed at the cell surface as a type I transmembrane precursor, proHB-EGF (Figure 2). The extracellular portion of proHB-EGF contains a bioactive EGF-like sequence; the intracellular portion, consisting of 24 amino acids, interacts with transcriptional repressors [12, 13]. ProHB-EGF is cleaved at a juxtamembrane site by activated metalloproteases, yielding a soluble growth factor derived from the extracellular domain and a carboxyl-terminal fragment containing the transmembrane and cytoplasmic segments (HB-EGF-CTF).

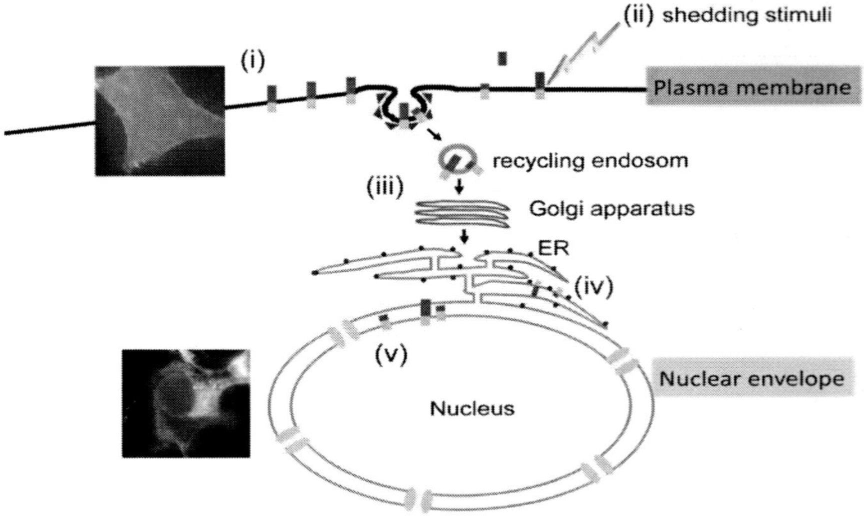

Figure 2. Intracellular trafficking pathways of HB-EGF. (i) proHB-EGF is predominantly expressed on the cell surface. (ii) Upon exposure to shedding stimuli, proHB-EGF is cleaved to yield soluble HB-EGF and membrane-anchored carboxyl-terminal fragment (HB-EGF-CTF), potentially altering the equilibrium between endocytosis and recycling. (iii) HB-EGF-CTF and remnant proHB-EGF may undergo retrograde transport to the Golgi apparatus via recycling endosomes, followed by (iv) targeting to the ER. The ER retrieval signal may be activated in response to shedding stimuli. (v) Subsequently, ER-localized membrane-anchored HB-EGF (either proHB-EGF or HB-EGF-CTF) diffuses or is actively transported to the INM via the NPC, and is ultimately tethered at the INM.

This process, termed ectodomain shedding, can be stimulated by various physiological and pharmacological agonists, including 12-*0*-tetradecanoylphorbol-13-acetate (TPA), calcium ionophores, and ligands of G protein–coupled receptors [14-16]. I showed previously that in addition to the extracellular EGF-like growth factor domain, which mediates a well-characterized signaling pathway, the remainder of the protein is also involved in intracellular signaling. Membrane-anchored HB-EGF, comprising both unshed proHB-EGF and HB-EGF-CTF, migrates from the plasma membrane to the ER and INM (Figure 3). Once the protein is localized to the INM, the cytoplasmic domain of HB-EGF faces the nucleoplasm and directly regulates gene expression [12, 13]. Furthermore, proHB-EGF expressed on the plasma membrane also functions as the sole cellular receptor for diphtheria toxin [17-19]. Binding of diphtheria toxin to proHB-EGF induces endocytosis of the proHB-EGF/toxin complex via clathrin-coated pits, followed by transport to the lysosome; subsequently, the toxin is released into the cytoplasm, where it inhibits protein synthesis [20, 21].

II. Protein Translocation from the Plasma Membrane to the Nucleus

The nucleus is surrounded by the nuclear envelope, a double lipid bilayer consisting of the INM and outer nuclear membrane (ONM). The membranes of the nuclear envelope form a non-permeable barrier; intracellular transport of macromolecules between the nucleus and cytoplasm takes place through the nuclear pore complexes (NPCs), which permit passive diffusion of molecules smaller than 40 kD and also support active and receptor-mediated transport. The INM and ONM are continuous at the NPC, but their protein compositions are radically different. Likewise, the ONM is continuous with the ER, but these two compartments also have distinct protein compositions [22, 23]. Integral membrane proteins targeted to the INM move from the ONM to the INM through the NPCs.

Recent studies have shown that many cell surface–associated macromolecules, ranging from receptor tyrosine kinases to cell-adhesion molecules, can traffic to the nuclear compartments including both the nucleoplasm and nuclear envelope. The INM and NPC play important and specific functions in genome organization, gene expression, DNA damage responses, and other processes [24, 25].

Nuclear targeting of cell-surface integral membrane proteins proceeds via three separate pathways (Figure 4). The first of these is targeting of intact polypeptides to the nucleoplasm (Figure 4, A). The nuclear localization of EGFR family members was first observed over 20 years ago [26-28]. Subsequently, nuclear localization of multiple cell-surface integral membrane proteins, including EGFR, ErbB-2, and FGF receptor, was reported by multiple groups, although it remains mysterious how membrane proteins can be localized in the nucleoplasm [29-32]. Recently, the underlying molecular mechanism has been partially revealed for EGFR, but not for other proteins [33-35].

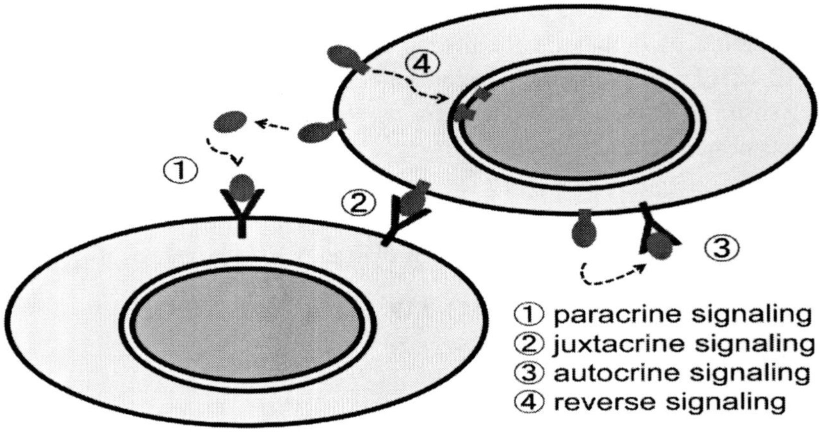

Figure 3. HB-EGF signaling pathways. As with other EGFR ligands, the EGF-like growth factor domain of HB-EGF is sufficient to elicit EGFR phosphorylation via autocrine, juxtacrine, and paracrine signaling pathways. Ectodomain shedding stimuli also appear to initiate another signaling pathway, in which the cytoplasmic domain of HB-EGF suppresses transcriptional repression in the HB-EGF–expressing cell via direct interactions with transcriptional repressors. A growing body of evidence indicates that membrane-integrated ligands such as TNF-α or ephrin can transmit signals into ligand-bearing cells. In these signaling pathways, referred to as 'reverse signaling', known membrane-bound ligands also function as receptors to trigger intracellular signaling events in ligand-bearing cells, thereby modifying their behavior. Shedding stimuli trigger intracellular signaling by HB-EGF and amphiregulin; thus, these pathways are examples of reverse signaling.

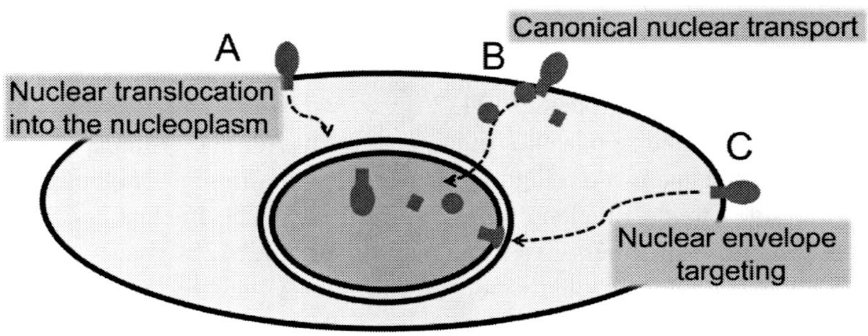

Figure 4. Intracellular protein translocation from the cell surface to the nucleus. A, unconventional nuclear transport from the plasma membrane to the nucleus. B. conventional nuclear transport. C, nuclear envelope targeting via membrane trafficking.

The functions of nuclear-localized plasma membrane proteins have been intensively studied under normal and perturbed conditions; these studies have been summarized in several excellent reviews [29-32]. The second pathway utilizes the canonical nuclear transport pathways such as that mediated by the importin β family (Figure 4, B). Some plasma membrane proteins, such as cadherin family and Notch proteins, are released by γ-secretase–mediated proteolysis, and then targeted to the nucleus as soluble proteins via these canonical pathways [36-39]. The third pathway is ‘nuclear envelope targeting’ via membrane trafficking (Figure 4, C), first demonstrated for HB-EGF and amphiregulin [9-11]. Some proteins are trafficked to the nucleus through a retrograde pathway from the plasma membrane to the ER, and then translocated to the INM. This pathway may be shared by nucleoplasm-targeted proteins such as EGFR, which is released from the membrane after INM targeting [34, 35]. In addition to proteins targeted specifically to the nuclear envelope from the plasma membrane, multiple plasma membrane proteins have been found in the ER or nuclear envelope, including the inositol 1,4,5-trisphopate (InsP3) receptor, NMDA receptor, and several ion-channel proteins including a large conductance nonselective cation channel and the potassium channel Kv10.1 [40-45]. In particular, Kv10.1 is targeted from the plasma membrane to the INM.

III. Possibilities for Drug Delivery

HB-EGF is a natural receptor for diphtheria toxin, which is often used in targeted toxins therapies [46, 47]. Moreover, HB-EGF is expressed in various cancers, including ovarian and breast tumors, and a clinical trial of HB-EGF as a cancer therapy is currently underway [48]. Because cells are compartmentalized into membrane-bound organelles, which are essential for the spatial restriction of specific physiological activities, drugs must be delivered to the correct intracellular compartments at the correct times in order to function appropriately and avoid degradation.

At steady state, HB-EGF is expressed on the cell surface, and it undergoes regulated translocation into a wide range of intracellular compartments under certain conditions. Therefore, uncovering the molecular mechanism of HB-EGF intracellular trafficking should enable development of novel modes of drug delivery.

Acknowledgments

This work was supported by Grants-in-Aid for Scientific Research from the Japan Society for the Promotion of Science, and by a Grant-in-Aid for Scientific Research on Innovative Areas from the Ministry of Education, Culture, Sports, Science and Technology of Japan. A part of this study was performed as part of a joint research program with Wako Pure Chemical Industries Ltd.

References

[1] Besner, G., Higashiyama, S. & Klagsbrun, M. (1990). Isolation and characterization of a macrophage-derived heparin-binding growth factor. *Cell Regul.,* 1, 811-819.

[2] Higashiyama, S., Abraham, J. A., Miller, J., Fiddes, J. C. & Klagsbrun, M. (1991). A heparin-binding growth factor secreted by macrophage-like cells that is related to EGF. *Science,* 251, 936-939.

[3] Higashiyama, S., Lau, K., Besner, G. E., Abraham, J. A. & Klagsbrun, M. (1992). Structure of heparin-binding EGF-like growth factor. Multiple forms, primary structure, and glycosylation of the mature protein. *J. Biol. Chem.,* 267, 6205-1622.

[4] Davis-Fleischer, K. M. & Besner, G. E. (1998). Structure and function of heparin-binding EGF-like growth factor (HB-EGF). *Front Biosci.,* 3, d288-299.

[5] Vinante, F. & Rigo, A. (2013). Heparin-binding epidermal growth factor-like growth factor/diphtheria toxin receptor in normal and neoplastic hematopoiesis. *Toxins (Basel).,* 5, 1180-1201.

[6] Bonifacino, J. S. & Rojas, R. (2006). *Nature Rev. Mol. Cell Biol.,* 7, 568-579.

[7] Johannes, L. & Popoff, V. (2008). Tracing the retrograde route in protein trafficking. Cell, 135, 1175-1187.

[8] Taguchi, T. (2013). Emerging roles of recycling endosomes. *J. Biochem.,* 153, 505-510.

[9] Hieda, M., Isokane, M., Koizumi, M., Higashi, C., Tachibana,T., Shudou, M., Tomohiko, T., Hieda, Y. & Higashiyama, S. (2008). Membrane-anchored growth factor, HB-EGF, on the cell surface targeted to the inner nuclear membrane. *J. Cell Biol.*, 180, 763-769.

[10] Isokane, M., Hieda, M., Hirakawa, S., Shudou, M., Nakashiro, K., Hashimoto, K., Hamakawa, H. & Higashiyama, S. (2008). Plasma-membrane-anchored growth factor pro-amphiregulin binds A-type lamin and regulates global ranscription. J. Cell Sci., 121, 3608-3018.

[11] Hieda, M., Koizumi, M., Higashi, C., Tachibana, T., Taguchi, T. & Higashiyama, S. (2012). The cytoplasmic tail of heparin-binding EGF-like growth factor regulates bidirectional intracellular trafficking between the plasma membrane and ER. *FEBS Open Bio.,* 2, 339-344.

[12] Nanba, D., Mammoto, A., Hashimoto, K. & Higashiyama, S. (2003). Proteolytic release of the carboxy-terminal fragment of proHB-EGF causes nuclear export of PLZF. *J. Cell Biol.,* 163, 489-502.

[13] Kinugasa, Y., Hieda, M., Hori, M. & Higashiyama, S. (2007). The carboxyl-terminal fragment of proHB-EGF reversed Bcl6-mediated gene repression. *J. Biol. Chem.,* 282, 14797-14806.

[14] Goishi, K., Higashiyama, S., Klagsbrun, M., Nakano, N., Umata, T., Ishikawa, M., Mekada, E. & Taniguchi, N. (1995). Phorbol ester induces the rapid processing of cell surface heparin-binding EGF-like growth factor: conversion from juxtacrine to paracrine growth factor activity. *Mol. Biol. Cell,* 6, 967-980.

[15] Dethlefsen, S. M., Raab, G., Moses, M. A., Adam, R. M., Klagsbrun, M. & Freeman, M. R. (1998). Extracellular calcium influx stimulates metalloproteinase cleavage and secretion of heparin-binding EGF-like growth factor independently of protein kinase *C. J. Cell. Biochem.,* 69, 143-153.

[16] Prenzel, N., Zwick, E., Daub, H., Leserer, M., Abraham, R., Wallasch, C. & Ullrich, A. (1999). EGF receptor transactivation by G-protein-coupled receptors requires metalloproteinase cleavage of proHB-EGF. *Nature,* 402, 884-888.

[17] Naglich, J. G., Metherall, J. E., Russell, D. W. & Eidels, L. (1992). Expression cloning of a diphtheria toxin receptor: identity with a heparin-binding EGF-like growth factor precursor. *Cell,* 69, 1051-1061.

[18] Iwamoto, R., Higashiyama, S., Mitamura, T., Taniguchi, N., Klagsbrun, M. & Mekada, E. (1994). Heparin-binding EGF-like growth factor, which acts as the diphtheria toxin receptor, forms a complex with membrane protein DRAP27/CD9, which up-regulates functional receptors anddiphtheria toxin sensitivity. *EMBO J.,* 13, 2322-2330.

[19] Mitamura, T., Iwamoto, R., Umata, T., Yomo, T., Urabe, I., Tsuneoka, M. & Mekada, E. (1992). The 27-kD diphtheria toxin receptor-associated protein (DRAP27) from vero cells is the monkey homologue

of human CD9 antigen: expression of DRAP27 elevates the number o diphtheria toxinreceptors on toxin-sensitive cells. *J Cell Biol.* 118, 1389-1399.

[20] Morris, R. E., Gerstein, A. S., Bonventre, P. F. & Saelinger, C. B. (1985). Receptor-mediated entry of diphtheria toxin into monkey kidney (Vero) cells: electron microscopic evaluation. *Infect Immun.,* 50, 721-727.

[21] Chang, M. P., Bramhall, J., Graves, S., Bonavida, B. & Wisnieski, B. J. (1989). Internucleosomal DNA cleavage precedes diphtheria toxin-induced cytolysis. Evidence that cell lysis is not a simple consequence of translation inhibition. J. Biol. Chem., 264, 15261-15267.

[22] Schirmer, E. C. & Gerace, L. (2005). The nuclear membrane proteome: extending the envelope. *Trends Biochem Sci.,* 30, 551-558.

[23] Schirmer, E. C. & Foisner, R. (2007). Proteins that associate with lamins: many faces, many functions. *Exp. Cell Res.,* 313, 2167-2179.

[24] Akhtar, A. & Gasser, S, M. (2007). The nuclear envelope and transcriptional control. *Nat. Rev. Genet.,* 8, 507-517.

[25] Brown, C. R. & Silver, P. A. (2007). Transcriptional regulation at the nuclear pore complex. *Curr. Opin. Genet. Dev.,* 17, 100-106.

[26] Raper, S. E., Burwen, S. J., Barker, M. E. & Jones, A. L. (1987). Translocation of epidermal growth factor to the hepatocyte nucleus during rat liver regeneration. *Gastroenterology,* 92, 1243-1250.

[27] Kamio, T., Shigematsu, K., Sou, H., Kawai, K. & Tsuchiyama, H. (1990). Immunohistochemical expression of epidermal growth factor receptors in human adrenocortical carcinoma. *Hum. Pathol.,* 21, 277-282.

[28] Marti, U., Burwen, S. J., Wells, A., Barker, M. E., Huling, S., Feren, A. M. & Jones, A. L. (1991). Localization of epidermal growth factor receptor in hepatocyte nuclei. *Hepatology*, 13, 15-20.

[29] Wang, Y. N. & Hung, M. C. (2012). Nuclear functions and subcellular trafficking mechanisms of the epidermal growth factor receptor family. *Cell Biosci.,* 2, 13.

[30] Bryant, D. M., & Stow, J. L. (2005). Nuclear translocation of cell-surface receptors: lessons from fibroblast growth factor. *Traffic,* 10, 947-954.

[31] Lin, S.Y., Makino, K., Xia, W., Matin, A., Wen, Y., Kwong, K.Y, Bourguignon, L. & Hung, M.C. (2001). Nuclear localization of EGF receptor and its potential new role as a transcription factor. Nat. Cell Biol., 3,, 802-808.

[32] Carpenter, G. & Liao, H. J. (2013). Receptor tyrosine kinases in the nucleus. Cold Spring Harb. Perspect. Biol., 5, a008979.

[33] Liao, H. J. & Carpenter, G. (2007). Role of the Sec61 translocon in EGF receptor trafficking to the nucleus and gene expression. Mol. Biol. Cell., 18, 1064-1072.

[34] Wang, Y. N., Yamaguchi, H., Huo, L., Du, Y., Lee, H. J., Lee, H. H., Wang, H., Hsu, J. M. & Hung, M. C. (2010). The translocon Sec61beta localized in the inner nuclear membrane transports membrane-embedded EGF receptor to the nucleus. *J. Biol. Chem.,* 285, 38720-38729.

[35] Wang, Y. N., Wang, H., Yamaguchi, H., Lee, H. J., Lee, H. H. & Hung, M. C. (2010). MCCOPI-mediated retrograde trafficking from the Golgi to the ER regulates EGFR nuclear transport. *Biochem. Biophys. Res. Commun.,* 399, 498-504.

[36] Stoeck, A, Shang, L. & Dempsey, P. J. (2010). Sequential and gamma-secretase-dependent processing of the betacellulinprecursor generates a palmitoylated intracellular-domain fragment that inhibits cell growth. *J Cell Sci.,* 123, 2319-2331.

[37] Cavallaro, U. & Dejana, E. (2011). Adhesion molecule signalling: not always a sticky business. *Nature Rev. Mol. Cell Biol.,* 12, 189-197.

[38] Kopan, R. & Ilagan, M. X. (2009). The canonical Notch signaling pathway: unfolding the activation mechanism. *Cell,* 137, 216-233.

[39] Bray, S. J. (2006). Notch signalling: a simple pathway becomes complex. *Nat. Rev. Mol. Cell Biol.,* 7, 678-689.

[40] Mazzanti, M., Bustamante, J. O., Oberleithner, H. (2001). Electrical dimension of the nuclear envelope. *Physiol. Rev.,* 81, 1-19.

[41] Marchenko, S. M., Yarotskyy, V. V., Kovalenko, T. N., Kostyuk, P. G. & Thomas, R. C. (2005). Spontaneously active and InsP3-activated ion channels in cell nuclei from rat cerebellar Purkinje and granule neurones. *J. Physiol.,* 565, 897-910.

[42] Fedorenko, O., Yarotskyy, V., Duzhyy, D., Marchenko, S. (2010). The large-conductance ion channels in the nuclear envelope of central neurons. Pflugers. Arch., 460, 1045-1050.

[43] Chen, Y., Sánchez, A., Rubio, M.E., Kohl, T., Pardo, L.A., and Stühmer, W. (2011). Functional K(v)10.1 channels localize to the inner nuclear membrane. *PLoS One.* 6, e19257.

[44] Zito, E., Buono, M., Pepe, S., Settembre, C., Annunziata, I., Surace, E. M., Dierks, T., Monti, M., Cozzolino, M., Pucci, P., Ballabio, A. & Cosma, M. P. (2007). Sulfatase modifying factor 1 trafficking through

the cells: from endoplasmic reticulum to the endoplasmic reticulum. *EMBO J.,* 26, 2443-2453.

[45] Benlimame, N., Le, P. U. & Nabi, I. R. (1998). Localization of Autocrine Motility Factor Receptor to Caveolae and Clathrin-independent Internalization of Its Ligand to Smooth Endoplasmic Reticulum. *Mol. Biol. Cell,* 9, 1773–1178.

[46] Pastan, I,, Hassan, R., Fitzgerald, D. J. & Kreitman, R. J. (2006). Immunotoxin therapy of cancer. *Nat. Rev. Cancer*, 6, 559-565.

[47] Li, Y. M., Vallera, D. A. & Hall, W. A. (2013). Diphtheria toxin-based targeted toxin therapy for brain tumors. *J Neurooncol.* 114, 155-164.

[48] Yagi, H., Yotsumoto, F., Sonoda, K., Kuroki, M., Mekada, E. & Miyamoto, S. (2009). Synergistic anti-tumor effect of paclitaxel with CRM197, an inhibitor of HB-EGF, in ovarian cancer. *Int. J. Cancer,* 283, 26089-26097.

Index

C

D

H

I

J

K

L

P

R

S

T